Patterns of Cancer
in Five Continents

INTERNATIONAL AGENCY FOR RESEARCH ON CANCER

The International Agency for Research on Cancer (IARC) was established in 1965 by the World Health Assembly as an independently financed organization within the framework of the World Health Organization. The headquarters of the Agency are at Lyon, France.

The Agency conducts a programme of research concentrating particularly on the epidemiology of cancer and the study of potential carcinogens in the human environment. Its field studies are supplemented by biological and chemical research carried out in the Agency's laboratories in Lyon and, through collaborative research agreements, in national research institutions in many countries. The Agency also conducts a programme for the education and training of personnel for cancer research.

The publications of the Agency are intended to contribute to the dissemination of authoritative information on different aspects of cancer research. A complete list is printed at the back of this volume.

INTERNATIONAL ASSOCIATION OF CANCER REGISTRIES

The International Association of Cancer Registries (IACR) was created in 1970, following a decision taken during the Ninth International Cancer Congress held in Tokyo, Japan in 1966. The Association is a voluntary non-governmental organization in official relations with WHO representing the scientific and professional interests of cancer registries, with members interested in the development and application of cancer registration and morbidity survey techniques to studies of well-defined populations.

The constitution provides for a Governing Body composed of a President, General Secretary, Deputy Secretary and eight regional representatives. From 1973 the IARC has provided a secretariat for the Association with the primary functions of organizing meetings and coordinating scientific studies.

WORLD HEALTH ORGANIZATION

INTERNATIONAL AGENCY FOR RESEARCH ON CANCER

and

INTERNATIONAL ASSOCIATION OF CANCER REGISTRIES

Patterns of Cancer in Five Continents

Editors

S. L. Whelan, D.M. Parkin and E. Masuyer

In collaboration with M. Smans

IARC Scientific Publications No. 102

International Agency for Research on Cancer

Lyon, 1990

Published by the International Agency for Research on Cancer,
150 cours Albert Thomas, 69372 Lyon Cedex 08, France

ISBN 92 832 2102 8

ISSN 0300-5085

Printed in France

Contents

Foreword vii

Maps viii

List of contributors xii

Introduction 1

Notes on the data 4

Part I. Histograms depicting rates of cancer age-standardized
to the 'world' population by site and sex 7

Part II. Pie diagrams showing relative frequencies of the
ten top-ranking cancer sites 55

Part III. Graphs of age-specific cancer incidence rates, by
site and sex 111

Cancer Incidence in Five Continents

This series of volumes presents, in each volume, a worldwide compilation of reliable cancer incidence data. The first two of the series were published by UICC in 1966 and 1970, and the subsequent volumes by IARC in collaboration with the International Association of Cancer Registries.

Volume I

Doll R., Payne P. & Waterhouse, J., eds (1966) *Cancer Incidence in Five Continents,* Vol. I. A technical report, UICC, Berlin, Springer Verlag (out of print)

Volume II

Doll R., Muir C. & Waterhouse, J., eds (1970) *Cancer Incidence in Five Continents,* Vol. II. Geneva, UICC (out of print)

Volume III

Waterhouse J., Muir C.S., Correa P. & Powell, J., eds (1976) *Cancer Incidence in Five Continents,* Vol. III. (IARC Scientific Publications No. 15), Lyon, International Agency for Research on Cancer (out of print)

Volume IV

Waterhouse J., Muir C., Shanmugaratnam K. & Powell, J., eds (1982) *Cancer Incidence in Five Continents,* Vol. IV. (IARC Scientific Publications No. 42), Lyon, International Agency for Research on Cancer (out of print)

Volume V

Muir C., Waterhouse J., Mack T., Powell J. & Whelan S., eds (1987) *Cancer Incidence in Five Continents,* Vol. V. (IARC Scientific Publications No. 88), Lyon, International Agency for Research on Cancer

Foreword

The study of geographical and ethnic variation in cancer occurrence has proved of great value in providing clues to the aetiology of cancer, and in estimating the proportion of different cancers likely to be due to 'environmental' differences between populations. The International Agency for Research on Cancer, in association with the International Association of Cancer Registries, publishes data from cancer registries around the world in the series of volumes *Cancer Incidence in Five Continents*. These have provided an invaluable and widely used resource for cancer researchers interested in evaluating the relative importance of environmental factors in the risk of different cancers.

Volume V of the series, published in 1987, included results from cancer registries covering 137 populations in 36 countries. In the present volume, the same data are represented in the form of diagrams — as histograms, pie charts and line-graphs. The intention is to permit a more rapid perception of the worldwide patterns and range in incidence for the different sites of cancer.

The contributing cancer registries are to be congratulated on their continuing efforts to provide reliable and accurate data on cancer incidence (sometimes in difficult local circumstances) which allow international comparative studies to be made.

Lorenzo Tomatis, M.D.
Director, IARC

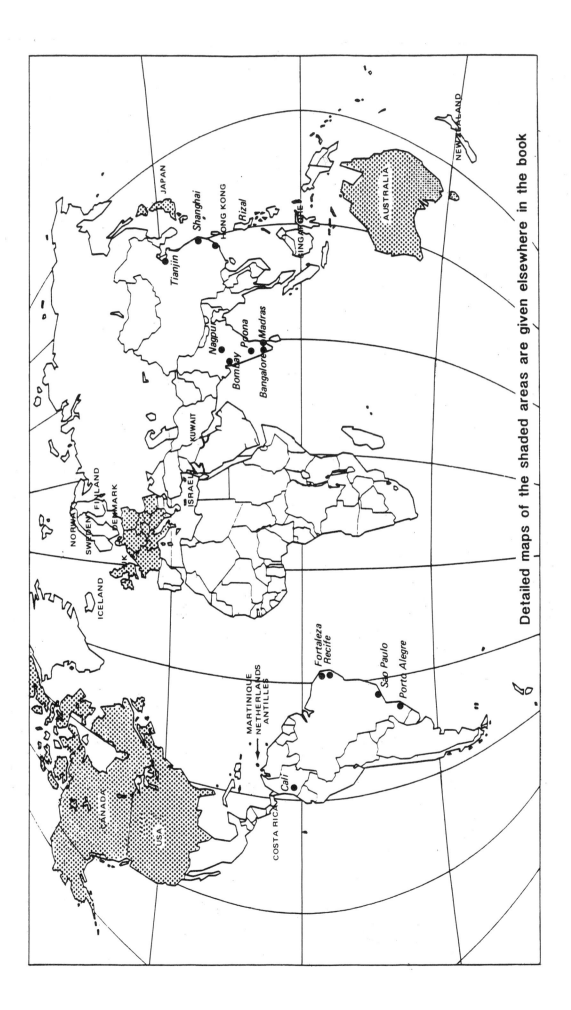

Detailed maps of the shaded areas are given elsewhere in the book

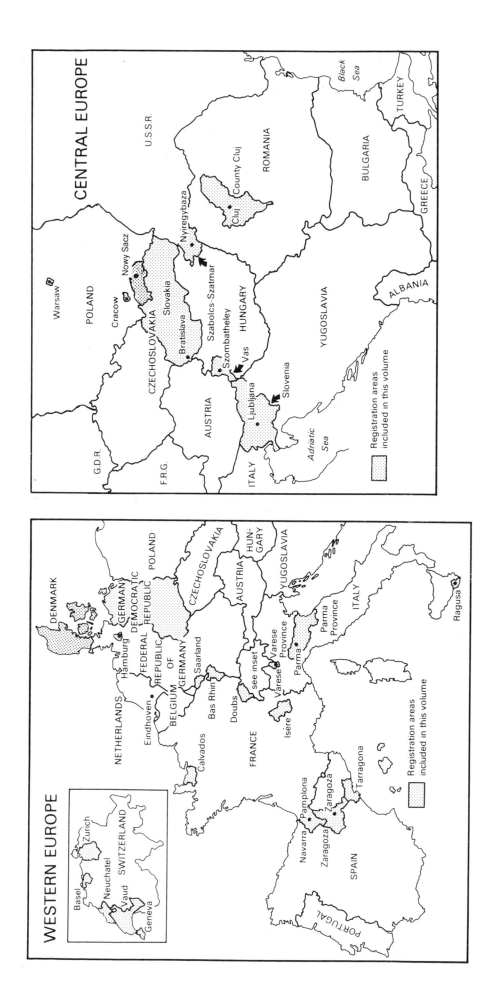

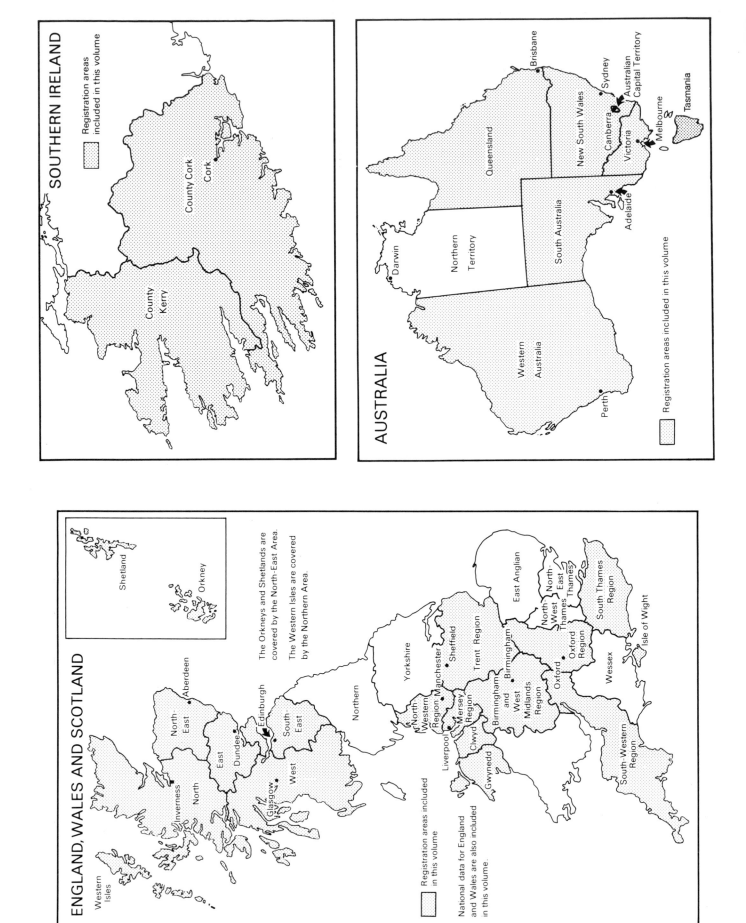

SOUTHERN IRELAND

Registration areas included in this volume

County Cork

Cork

County Kerry

AUSTRALIA

Brisbane

Queensland

Northern Territory

South Australia

New South Wales

Sydney

Canberra — Australian Capital Territory

Victoria — Melbourne

Tasmania

Adelaide

Darwin

Western Australia

Perth

Registration areas included in this volume

ENGLAND, WALES AND SCOTLAND

Shetland

Orkney

The Orkneys and Shetlands are covered by the North-East Area.

The Western Isles are covered by the Northern Area.

Western Isles

Aberdeen

North-East

Edinburgh

South-East

Inverness

North

East

Dundee

West

Glasgow

Yorkshire

Northern

North Western Region

Manchester

Liverpool

Mersey Region

Sheffield

Trent Region

Clwyd

Gwynedd

Birmingham and West Midlands Region

Birmingham

East Anglian

North West Thames

North East Thames

Oxford

Oxford Region

South Thames Region

Wessex

Isle of Wight

South-Western Region

Registration areas included in this volume

National data for England and Wales are also included in this volume.

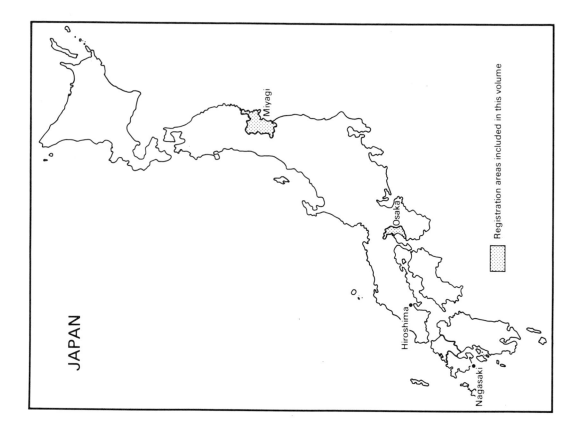

JAPAN

Miyagi

Osaka

Hiroshima

Nagasaki

Registration areas included in this volume

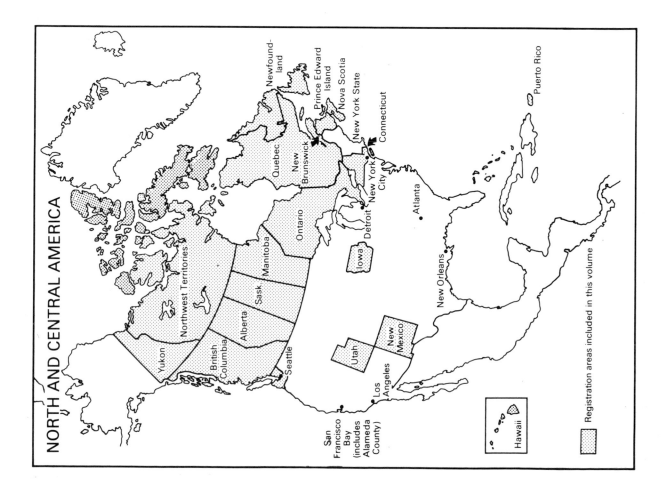

NORTH AND CENTRAL AMERICA

Newfound-
land

Prince Edward
Island

Nova Scotia

New York State

Connecticut

Quebec

New
Brunswick

New York
City

Ontario

Detroit

Iowa

Atlanta

Manitoba

New Orleans

Sask.

New
Mexico

Alberta

Utah

British
Columbia

Los
Angeles

Northwest Territories

Seattle

Yukon

San
Francisco
Bay
(includes
Alameda
County)

Puerto Rico

Hawaii

Registration areas included in this volume

Contributors

Note : The contributors to *Cancer Incidence in Five Continents,* Volume V, whose data are used in this volume are listed below.

CENTRAL & SOUTH AMERICA

Brazil, Fortaleza

Registro de Cancer do Ceará (Cancer Registry of Ceará), Rua Papi Junior, 1222 - Rodolfo Teofilo, 60430 Fortaleza-Ceará, Brazil. Tel : (085) 223 28 00
Marcelo Gurgel C. Silva, Haroldo Gondim Juaçaba, Dalgimar Beserra Meneses, José Gomes Bezerra Filho

Brazil, Pernambuco, Recife

Registro de Cancer de Pernambuco (Cancer Registry of Pernambuco), Faculdade de Medicina da Universidade Federal de Pernambuco, Cidade Universitaria, 50730 - Recife, Pernambuco, Brazil. Tel : (081) 235 3380
Manoel Ricardo da Costa Carvalho, Adonis Carvalho, Otacilio Araújo da Silva, Vital Lira, Theonas Pimentel Fernandes Lima, Gicelia Valença de Lira

Brazil, Porto Alegre

Registro de Cancer de Porto Alegre (Cancer Registry of Porto Alegre), Av. Washington Luiz, 868, 90310 - Porto Alegre - RS, Brazil. Tel : (0512) 26 3689
L. Borges Barcelos

Brazil, São Paulo

São Paulo Cancer Registry, Av. Dr Arnaldo, 715, 01255 São Paulo - SP, Brazil. Tel : (011) 278 8811
A.P. Mirra, J.M.P. de Souza, J.P.A. de Freitas, C. Marigo, S.L. Gotlieb, R. Laurenti, E.F. Pastorelo

Colombia, Cali

Registro de Cancer de Cali (Cancer Registry of Cali), Department of Pathology, University of Valle, Sede San Fernando, Apartado Aereo 25360, Cali, Colombia. Tel : 582110 Ext. 30
Carlos Cuello, Tito Collazos, Pelayo Correa, William Haenszel

Costa Rica

Registro Nacional de Tumores (Cancer Registry of Costa Rica), Departamento de Estadistica, Unidad Sectorial de Planification, Ministerio de Salud, San José, Republica de Costa Rica
Luzmilda Lopez Guzman, Georgina Muñoz Leiva, Bernardo Moreyra Moreyra, Wilder Thorpe Calderon, Ligia Valladares Zuchini, Margarita Marenco Ovares

France, Martinique

Registre du Cancer de la Martinique (Cancer Registry of Martinique), A.M.R.E.C., Centre Hospitalier de Fort-de-France, B.P. 993, 97247 Fort-de-France Cedex, Martinique, France. Tel : 73 13 38, Telex : 029519
M. Fagart, H. Azaloux, R. Salamon, P. Escarmant, A. Saint-Cyr, G. le Mab

Netherlands Antilles (less Aruba)

Netherlands Antilles Cancer Registry, c/o Stan C. Freni, MD, National Center for Toxicological Research, Biometry Staff, Jefferson, Arkansas 72079, USA.
Stan C. Freni

USA, Puerto Rico

Central Cancer Registry of Puerto Rico, Department of Health, P.O. Box 9342, Santurce, Puerto Rico 00908, USA. Tel : (809) 751 6160
Isidro Martinez, Raquel Torres, Lucy Echevarría, Nadgie E. Zea, Juana R. Marrero, Nieves E. Perez, Maria M. Rivera

NORTH AMERICA

Canada

National Cancer Incidence Reporting System, Health Division, Statistics Canada, R.H. Coats Building, Tunney's Pasture, Ottawa, Ontario, Canada K1A OT6. Tel : (613) 995 9593, Telex : 053 3585

Anna Brancker, Leslie Gaudette, Diane Badger,
Mike Gunville, Peter Lim

Canada, Alberta
Alberta Cancer Registry, Department of
Epidemiology & Preventive Oncology, Alberta
Cancer Board, 6th Floor, Capital Place, 9707 -
110 Street, Canada T5K 2L9. Tel : (403) 482-9370,
Fax : 488-7809
G.B. Hill, M. Koch, S. Huchcroft, J. Hanson,
M. Raphael, H. Gaedke

Canada, British Columbia
British Columbia Cancer Registry, Cancer Control
Agency of British Columbia, 600 West 10th
Avenue, Vancouver, British Columbia, Canada
V5Z 4E6. Tel : (604) 877 6000, Telex : 04-507648
D.A. Boyes, P. Hayles, M. McBride, L. Donaldson,
H. Hersom

Canada, Manitoba
Central Cancer Registry, Manitoba Cancer
Treatment & Research Foundation, 100 Olivia
Street, Winnipeg, Manitoba, Canada R3E OV9.
Tel : (204) 787 2157, (204) 787 2266
H. Schipper, L.G. Israels, N.W. Choi, N. Nelson,
J. Ediger, B. Wingert

Canada, New Brunswick
New Brunswick Provincial Tumour Registry, Saint
John Regional Hospital, Saint John, New
Brunswick, P.O. Box 2100, Canada E2L 4L2.
Tel : (506) 648 6871
Dorothy Robb, G.D. Smith, R. Nimmagadda

Canada, Nova Scotia
Cancer Registry, Province of Nova Scotia, Cancer
Treatment & Research Foundation of Nova Scotia,
5820 University Avenue, Halifax, Nova Scotia,
Canada B3H 1V7. Tel : (902) 428-4209
D.H. Thomson, Thelma Croucher, Jean James

Canada, Prince Edward Island
Department of Health & Social Services, Oncology
Division, P.O. Box 2000, Charlottetown, Prince
Edward Island, Canada C1A 7N8.
Tel : (902) 892 5471
D.E. Dryer, W.T. Hooper, C. McAleer

Canada, Newfoundland
The Newfoundland Cancer Treatment & Research
Foundation, Provincial Tumor Registry, 25
Kenmount Road, St. John's, Newfoundland, Canada
A1B 1W1. Tel : (709) 753 2599
Donna Ball, S. Buehler

Canada, Northwest Territories & Yukon
Northwest Territories Cancer Registry, Department
of Health, Government of the NWT, Box 1320,
Yellowknife, North West Territories, Canada

X1A 2L9. Tel : (403) 920 6280, Telex : 034 45506
Luis Barreto, Leo Stec, Sharon Freitag, J. Nundarao

Canada, Ontario
Ontario Cancer Registry, Ontario Cancer Treatment
& Research Foundation, 7 Overlea Boulevard,
Toronto, Ontario, Canada M4H 1A8. Tel : (416)
423 4240
D. Dale, M. Nemes, H. Weir, J. Chin,
J. Gangadeen, J. Hum

Canada, Quebec
Fichier des Tumeurs du Québec, (Quebec Cancer
Registry), Ministère de la Santé et des Services
Sociaux, 1075, chemin Ste-Foy, 3e étage, Québec
(Québec), Canada G1S 2M1. Tel : (418) 643 9936
Guy Paul Sanscartier, Michel Beaupré, Jeanne
Bourdages, Clément Jean, Michel St-Amour

Canada, Saskatchewan
Saskatchewan Cancer Foundation, 2631-28th
Avenue, Suite 400, Regina, Saskatchewan, Canada
S4S 6X3. Tel : (306) 585 1831, Fax : (306) 584 2733
D.J. Klaassen, H.G. Whiston, D.L. Robson

USA, California, Alameda County
Bay Area Resource for Cancer Control, Northern
California Cancer Center, 1420 Harbor Bay
Parkway, Suite 260, Alameda, CA 94501-7080, USA.
Tel : (415) 748 6111, Fax : (415) 748 6118
Dee W. West, Lilia O'Connor, Helen Sanderson,
Thomas E. Davis, Donald F. Austin, Kay Bragg

USA, California, San Francisco Bay Area
Bay Area Resource for Cancer Control, Northern
California Cancer Center, 1420 Harbor Bay
Parkway, Suite 260, Alameda, CA 94501, USA.
Tel : (415) 748 6111
Dee W. West, Lilia O'Connor, Helen Sanderson,
Thomas E. Davis, Donald F. Austin, Kay Bragg

USA, California, Los Angeles County
Los Angeles County Cancer Surveillance Program,
University of Southern California, 1721 Griffin
Ave., Room 209, Los Angeles, California 90031,
USA. Tel : (213) 224 5190, Fax : (213) 224 5346
Thomas M. Mack, Herman R. Menck, Judith
R. Boone, Jean L. Torrance, Cynthia L. Conant

USA, Connecticut
Connecticut Tumor Registry, Connecticut
Department of Health Services, 150 Washington
Street, Hartford, Connecticut 06106, USA. Tel :
(203) 566 3975
John T. Flannery, Dwight T. Janerich,
Joan M. Gervais

USA, Georgia, Atlanta
Georgia Center for Cancer Statistics, Emory

University School of Medicine, 1599 Clifton Road, N.E., Atlanta, GA 30329, USA.
Tel: (404) 727 8720
Ray Greenberg, Jonathan Liff

USA, Iowa
State Health Registry of Iowa, Epidemiology Research Center, The University of Iowa, S.100 Westlawn, Iowa City, Iowa 52242, USA.
Tel: (319) 335 8609
Peter Isaacson, Charles Platz, Kathleen McKeen

USA, Louisiana, New Orleans
Louisiana Tumor Registry, DHHR Office of Preventive and Public Health Service, 325 Loyola Avenue, Room 305, New Orleans, LA 70112, USA.
Tel: (504) 568 2616
Jean F. Craig, Pelayo Correa, Vivien W. Chen

USA, Michigan, Detroit
Metropolitan Detroit Cancer Surveillance System, Division of Epidemiology, The Michigan Cancer Foundation, 110 E. Warren Ave., Detroit, Michigan 48201, USA. Tel: (313) 833 0710
G. Marie Swanson, William A. Satariano, Ann G. Schwartz, Joanne Harris, Michael G. Baracy

USA, New Mexico
New Mexico Tumor Registry, University of New Mexico Medical Center, 900 Camino de Salud NE, Albuquerque, NM 87131, USA.
Tel: (505) 277 5541
Charles Key, Mary Lerchen

USA, New York
New York State Cancer Registry, Bureau of Cancer Epidemiology, New York State Department of Health, Corning Tower, Room 565, Albany, NY 12237, USA. Tel: (518) 474 2255
W.S. Burnett, M.B. Hoff, P.E. Wolfgang, P.C. Masca, J. Mikl

USA, Utah
Utah Cancer Registry, 420 Chipeta Way, Suite 190, Salt Lake City, Utah 84108, USA.
Tel: (801) 581 5270
Dee W. West, R. Dibble, C. Davis

USA, Washington, Seattle
Cancer Surveillance System of Western Washington, The Fred Hutchinson Cancer Research Center, 1124 Columbia Street, Seattle, WA 98104, USA.
Tel: (206) 467 5000
D.B. Thomas, M. Potts, J. Chu

ASIA

China, Shanghai
Shanghai Cancer Registry, Shanghai Cancer Institute, 2200 Xie Tu Road, Shanghai 200032, People's Republic of China. Tel: 315360,
Telex: 33325 SFMC CN
Gao Yu-Tang, Jin Fan

China, Tianjin
Tianjin Cancer Registry, Tianjin Cancer Institute, Huan Hu Xi Road, Ti-Yuan-Bei, Tianjin 300060, People's Republic of China.
Tianze Zhang, Qingsheng Wang, Xiuyun Bai, Feng Su, Zheng Yie, Sufen Dong

Hong Kong
Hong Kong Cancer Registry, Hospital Services Department, Institute of Radiology & Oncology, Queen Elizabeth Hospital, Wylie Road, Kowloon, Hong Kong. Tel: 3-7102255
J.H.C. Ho, K.K. Man, S.Y. Tsao, P.K. Chan

India, Bangalore
Population-Based Cancer Registry-Bangalore (Indian Council of Medical Research), Kidwai Memorial Institute of Oncology, Hosur Road, Bangalore - 560 029, India. Tel: 40245
M. Krishna Bhargava, A. Nandakumar, R. Ramachandra Reddy

India, Bombay
Bombay Cancer Registry, Indian Cancer Society, 74, Jerbai Wadia Road, Parel, Bombay 400 012, India. Tel: 4121519
D.J. Jussawala, B.B. Yeole, M.V. Natekar

India, Madras
Madras Metropolitan Tumour Registry, Cancer Institute, Adyar, Tamil Nadu, Madras 600 020, India. Tel: 412714
V. Shanta, Nirmala Chandrasekaran, C.K. Gajalakshmi

India, Nagpur
Nagpur Cancer Registry Division, Bombay Cancer Registry, Indian Cancer Society, 74 Jerbai Wadia Road, Parel, Bombay 400 012, India. Tel: 4121519
D.J. Jussawalla, N.K. Desmukh, B.B. Yeole, M.V. Natekar

India, Poona
Poona Cancer Registry Division, Bombay Cancer Registry, Indian Cancer Society, 74 Jerbai Wadia Road, Parel, Bombay 400 012, India. Tel: 4121519
D.J. Jussawala, N.K. Desmukh, B.B. Yeole, M.V. Natekar

Israel
Israel Cancer Registry, Ministry of Health, 20 King David Street, Jerusalem 91000, Israel.
Tel: 011-972-2-247172
Leah Katz, Ruth Steinitz, Tovah Sela, Rachel Alon, Marianne Neuman

Japan, Hiroshima City
Hiroshima-shi Ishikai Shuyo Tokei Iinkai
(Hiroshima City Medical Association Tumor
Statistics Committee), 5-2 Hijiyama Park, Minami-
ku, Hiroshima 732, Japan. Tel: 082-232-7321
*Yoshihiko Yamashita, Hisashi Oshiro, Sumio
Sugimoto, Tsutomu Yamamoto, Suminori Akiba,
Kiyohiko Mabuchi*

Japan, Miyagi Prefecture
Miyagi Prefectural Cancer Registry, c/o Miyagi
Cancer Society, Kamisugi 6-chome, Aoba-ku,
Sendai 980, Japan. Tel: 022-233-0241 Ext. 45
*Mitsuo Segi (deceased), Akira Takano, Yoshi Okuno,
Sadao Okitsu, Minoru Kurihara*

Japan, Nagasaki City
Nagasaki-City Tumor Registry, Radiation Effects
Research Foundation, 8-6 Nakagawa 1-chome,
Nagasaki City, Nagasaki-ken 850, Japan.
Tel: 0958-23-1121
*Takayoshi Ideka, Midori Soda, Issei Nishimori,
Yoshisada Shibata, Masayuki Terasaki*

Japan, Osaka Prefecture
Osaka-fu Gan-toroku Shitsu (Osaka Cancer
Registry), Dept. of Field Research, Center for
Adult Diseases, 1-3-3 Nakamichi, Higashinari-ku,
Osaka 537, Japan. Tel: 06-972-1181 Ext. 2284,
2378
*Isaburo Fujimoto, Aya Hanai, Tsuneaki Takashina,
Muneo Sugimoto, Masamune Nanba, Akio Mitsuhashi*

Kuwait
Kuwait Cancer Registry, Kuwait Cancer Control
Centre, P.O. Box 42262, 70653 Shuwaikh, Kuwait.
Tel: 810007, 849100,
Telex: 22729 HEALTH KT
*Y.T. Omar, Abdel Aziz S. Ismail, Mahdi Jaber
Abu-Tabikh*

Philippines, Rizal Province
Rizal Medical Center Cancer Registry, Rizal
Medical Center, Shaw Blvd., Pasig, Metromanila
3130, Philippines D.2801.
*Adriano V. Laudico, Divina B. Esteban,
Glicerio M. Bustamante, Clarita B. Farre,
Tomas P. Maramba, Jane C. Baltazar*

Singapore
Singapore Cancer Registry, c/o Department of
Pathology, National University Hospital, Lower
Kent Ridge Road, Singapore 0511.
Tel: 7786783, 779-5555
Telex: NUSBUR RS51112
K. Shanmugaratnam, H.P. Lee, N.E. Day

EUROPE

Czechoslovakia, Slovakia
Národný onkologický register SSR (National Cancer
Registry of Slovakia), Oncological Center, 812 32
Bratislava, Ul. Csl. armády 21, Czechoslovakia.
Tel: (07) 575 41
*Ivan Plesko, Elena Dimitrova, Jozef Somogyi,
Andrej Sesták, Vladimír Vlasák*

Denmark
Danish Cancer Registry, Rosenvaengets Hovedvej
35, Box 839, DK 2100 Copenhagen, Denmark.
Tel: 01-26 88 66, Fax: 01-26 00 90
O.M. Jensen, A. Prener, H.H. Storm

Federal Republic of Germany, Hamburg
Hamburgisches Krebsregister Gesundheitsbehörde
Hamburg (Cancer Registry of Hamburg), Postfach
2534, Tesdorpfstr. 8, 2000 Hamburg 13, Federal
Republic of Germany. Tel: (040) 44 19 5 285
*W. Thiele, B. Buchhofer, C. Baumgardt-Elms,
U. Haartje*

Federal Republic of Germany, Saarland
Krebsregister des Saarlandes (Cancer Registry of
Saarland), Statistisches Amt des Saarlandes,
Hardenbergstr. 3, Postfach 409, 6600 Saarbrücken,
Federal Republic of Germany. Tel: (681) 505-969,
Telex: 442 1371
H. Ziegler, Ch. Stegmaier

Finland
Suomen Syoparekisteri (Finnish Cancer Registry),
Liisankatu 21 B, SF-00170 Helsinki 17, Finland.
Tel: 358-0-176290
*E. Saxén, M. Hakama, T. Hakulinen, M. Lehtonen,
E. Pukkala, L. Teppo*

France, Bas-Rhin
Registre Bas-Rhinois des Cancers (Bas-Rhin Cancer
Registry), Faculté de Médecine, 67085 Strasbourg
Cédex, France. Tel: 88 36 57 88
P. Schaffer

France, Calvados
1. Registre des Cancers du Calvados (Cancer
   Registry of Calvados), Centre François Baclesse,
   Route de Lion-sur-Mer, 14021 Caen Cédex,
   France.
   J. Robillard, J. Mace-Lesech, J.S. Abbatucci

2. Registre spécialisé Digestif, Centre Hospitalo-
   Universitaire, 14040 Caen Cedex, France.
   Tel: 31 45 50 50
   M. Gignoux, L. Chérié-Challine, M.D. Pottier

France, Doubs
Registre des Tumeurs du Doubs (Cancer Registry
of Doubs), C.H.R. Jean Minjoz, 1 Boulevard

Fleming, 25030 Besançon Cedex, France.
Tel: 81 52 33 22,
Telex: SAMU BESANÇON 360 436 F.
Simon Schraub, André Oppermann, Martine Belon-Leneutre, Mariette Mercier, Pierre Bourgeois

France, Isère
Registre du Cancer de l'Isère (Isère Cancer Registry), 21 chemin des Sources, 38240 Meylan, France. Tel: 76 90 76 10
F. Ménégoz, J.M. Lutz, R. Schaerer

German Democratic Republic
Nationales Krebsregister und -statistik (National Cancer Registry and Statistics by the Central Institute of Cancer Research), Academy of Sciences of the GDR, Sterndamm 13, 1197 Berlin-Johannisthal, German Democratic Republic.
Tel: (2) 635 36 48
W.H. Mehnert, P. Bernstein, J.F. Haas, W. Staneczek

Hungary, County Szabolcs-Szatmar
Szabolcs-Szatmar megyei Tanacs Korhaza Megyei Onkologiai Gondozo (Cancer Registry of the County Szabolcs-Szatmar), County Hospital, Vörös Hadsereg 68, H-4401 Nyiregyhaza, Hungary.
Tel: (42) 12 222/600 Telex: 73 426
Lajos Juhasz, Erzsébet Melich, Borbala Gaspar

Hungary, County Vas
County Vas Cancer Registry, Hospital 'Markusovszky', Szombathely, Semmelweis u.2, H-9700 Hungary. Tel: (95) 11 503
Eszter Kocsis

Iceland
Icelandic Cancer Registry, Skogarhlid 8, Postbox 5420, 125 Reykjavik, Iceland.
Hrafn Tulinius, Olafur Bjarnason, Helgi Sigvaldason, Gudrun Bjarnadottir, Gudridur H. Olafsdottir, Torfi Bjarnason

Ireland, Southern
Southern Tumour Registry, Ardpatrick House, College Road, Cork, Ireland. Tel: (021) 507 384, Telex: 76050
J.W. Magner, C.T. Doyle, J.P. Corridan, Michael Crowley, Patricia Holmes, Mary Hand

Italy, Lombardy Region, Varese Province
Registro Tumori Lombardia (Provincia de Varese) (Lombardy Cancer Registry (Varese Province)), Istituto Nazionale per lo Studio e la Cura dei Tumori, Via Venezian, 1, 20133 Milano, Italy.
Tel: (02) 2366342, Telex: 33290 TUMIST I
Franco Berrino, Paolo Crosignani, Gemma Gatta, Maurizio Macaluso, Paola Pisani, Clotilde Vigano

Italy, Parma Province
Registro Tumori Della Provincia di Parma (Cancer Registry of Parma Province), Servizio di Oncologia, Via Gramsci, 14, 43100 Parma, Italy.
Tel: (0521) 96723/991811
G. Cocconi, A. Borrini, L. Serventi, M. Zatelli, V. De Lisi, G. Malmassari

Italy, Ragusa Province
Registro Tumori Ragusa (Ragusa Cancer Registry), Usl. n° 23, Ospedale G.B. Odierna, Piazza Igea 2, Ragusa CAP. 97100, Italy. Tel: 0932 48534
Luigi Dardanoni, Lorenzo Gafà, G. Pavone, M. La Rosa, R. Spampinato

Netherlands, Eindhoven
SOOZ/IKZ Cancer Registry, Fellenoordcomplex gebouw 11, Pastoor Peterstraat 114, 5612 LT Eindhoven, The Netherlands. Tel: 040 455 775
J.W.C. Coebergh, M. Crommelin, M. Verhagen-Teulings, D. Bakker, L.V.O. Heyden

Norway
Cancer Registry of Norway, Institute for Epidemiological Cancer Research, Montebello, N-0310 Oslo 3, Norway. Tel: 02 506050
Aage Andersen, Tove Dahl, Steinar Hansen, Froydis Langmark, Liv Lie, Steinar Thoresen

Poland, Cracow City
Rejestr Nowotworow Miasta Krakowa i Nowego Sacza (Cracow City and Nowy Sacz Cancer Registry), Institute of Oncology, ul. Garncarska 11, 31-115 Krakow, Poland. Tel: 29 90 00, Telex: 0325437 JOOK PL
J. Pawlega, A. Urbanska, Z. Aksamit, E. Podgorska

Poland, Nowy Sacz
Rejestr Nowotworow Miasta Krakowa i Nowego Sacza (Cracow City and Nowy Sacz Cancer Registry), Institute of Oncology, ul. Garncarska 11, 31-115 Krakow, Poland. Tel: 29 90 00, Telex: 0325437 JOOK PL
J. Pawlega, A. Urbanska, Z. Aksamit, E. Podgorska

Poland, Warsaw City
Rejestr Nowotworow m.st. Warszawy (Warsaw Cancer Registry), Cancer Center of the Maria Sklodowska-Curie Institute, Wawelska 15, 00-973 Warsaw, Poland. Tel: 23 31 79, Telex: 812704 INONK PL
Helena Gadomska, Maria Jeziorska, Maria Zwierko, Janina Jachimiak, Alina Kuss, Zofia Przybysz

Romania, County Cluj
Fisierul cancerului-judetul Cluj (Cluj County Cancer Registry), Oncological Institute of Cluj-Napoca, Department of Epidemiology & Statistics, Str. Republicii nr. 34-36, R-3400 Cluj Napoca,

Romania. Tel: (951) 1 83 61
Gh. Bolba, M. Dordea, M. Szöllës

Spain, Catalonia, Tarragona
Registro de Cancer de Tarragona (Tarragona
Cancer Registry), Associacio Espanyola Contra el
Cancer, Avda. Maria Cristina 54, 43002 Tarragona,
Catalonia, Spain. Tel: 77222221
*J. Borras, J. Galceran, J.Ll. Creus, F.X. Bosch, P.
Viladiu, M. Campillo*

Spain, Navarra
Registro de Tumores de Navarra (Navarra Cancer
Registry), Ciudadela, 5-1°, 31001 - Pamplona
(Navarra), Spain. Tel: (948) 22 11 89
*Nieves Ascunce Elizaga, Ma Eugenia Perez de
Rada, Nieves Navaridas Hueto*

Spain, Zaragoza
Registro del Cancer de Zaragoza (Cancer Registry
of Zaragoza), Sanidad de la Diputacion General de
Aragon, c/ Ramon y Cajal, 68, 50004 - Zaragoza,
Spain. Tel: (976) 44 20 22
*Antonio Zubiri, Pedro Mateo, Lourdes Zubiri,
Carmen Martos, Alberto Vergara, Pilar Moreo*

Sweden
Cancerregistret, The National Board of Health &
Welfare, S-106 30 Stockholm, Sweden.
Tel: (08) 783 30 00, Telex: 16773 NBHW S
Thomas Gunnarson, Jan Ericsson

Switzerland, Basel
Krebsregister Basel-Stadt und Basel-Land (Basel
Cancer Registry), Department of Pathology,
University of Basel, Schonbeinstrasse 40, CH-4003
Basel, Switzerland. Tel: (061) 252525
J. Torhorst, P. Hendriks, R. Dougoud, E. Perret

Switzerland, Geneva
Registre genevois des tumeurs (Geneva Cancer
Registry), 55, bd de la Cluse, CH-1205 Geneva 4,
Switzerland. Tel: (022) 29 10 11
L. Raymond, M. Obradovic, A. Hickson

Switzerland, Neuchâtel
Registre Neuchâtelois des Tumeurs (Neuchâtel
Cancer Registry), Les Cadolles 4, CH-2000
Neuchâtel, Switzerland. Tel: (038) 243015
S. Pellaux, A.M. Méan, R.P. Baumann

Switzerland, Vaud
Registre Vaudois des Tumeurs, (Cancer Registry of
Vaud), Institut Universitaire de Médecine Sociale et
Préventive, CHUV BH 06, CH-1011 Lausanne,
Switzerland. Tel: (021) 413909
*F. Levi, F. Gutzwiller, R. Alaili, S. Chapallaz,
H.L. Gay, A. Randriamiharisoa*

Switzerland, Zürich
Kantonalzürcherisches Krebsregister (Cancer Registry
of the Canton of Zurich), Institute of Pathology,
University Hospital, CH-8091 Zurich, Switzerland.
Tel: (01) 255 3368
J.R. Rüttner, G. Schüler, D. Marczinski, D. Schüler

**United Kingdom, England & Wales National
Cancer Registry**
Office of Population Censuses & Surveys, Medical
Statistics Division, St Catherine's House,
10 Kingsway, London WC2B 6JP, UK.
Tel: 071-242-0262
A.J. Swerdlow, F.L. Ashwood, J.E. Good

UK, Birmingham and West Midlands Region
Birmingham & West Midlands Regional Registry,
Queen Elizabeth Medical Centre, Birmingham B15
2TH, UK. Tel: 021-472 1311, Telex: 33 89 38
SPAPHYG
*J.A.H. Waterhouse, C.A. Roginski, M. Collier,
K. Hughes, J. Dansage, V. Wilkes*

UK, England, North Western Region
North Western Regional Cancer Registry, Christie
Hospital & Holt Radium Institute, Wilmslow Road,
Withington, Manchester M20 9BX, UK.
Tel: (061) 445 8123 Ext. 586
*A. Smith, R.T. Benn, V. Blair, J. Cook,
N. Willows, B. Feighan*

UK, England, Oxford Region
Oxford Cancer Registry, Oxford Regional Health
Authority, Old Road, Headington, Oxford
OX3 7LF, UK. Tel: (0865) 64861
C. Hunt, A. Barr, E. Rue

UK, England, South Thames Region
The Thames Cancer Registry, Clifton Avenue,
Belmont, Sutton, Surrey SM2 5PY, UK.
Tel: (081) 642 7692
R.G. Skeet, H. Thornton-Jones

UK, England, South Western Region
South Western RHA Cancer Registry, Records
Bureau, UTF House, 26 King Square, Bristol
BS2 8HY, UK.
P. Watts, J. Adams

UK, England, Trent Region
Trent Regional Cancer Registration Bureau, Trent
Regional Health Authority, Fulwood House, Old
Fulwood Road, Sheffield S10 3TH, UK. Tel:
(0742) 306511,
Telex: 547246 TRHAG
D.S. Maclean, I.M. Ainsworth, K. White

UK, England & Wales, Mersey Region
Mersey Regional Cancer Registry, Hamilton House,
24 Pall Mall, Liverpool L3 6AL, UK.

Tel: (051) 236 4620
M.V. Rivlin, S.M. Gravestock, R. Dee, D.N. Edwards (retd), E.M. McConnell (retd.)

UK, Scotland, Scottish Cancer Registry
Trinity Park House, South Trinity Road, Edinburgh EH5 3SQ, Scotland, UK.
Tel: (031) 552 6255
I.W. Kemp

UK, Scotland, East
Scotland-East Cancer Registry, P.O. Box 75, Vernonholme, Riverside Drive, Dundee DD1 9NL, Scotland, UK. Tel: (0382) 645151,
Fax: (0382) 69734
N. Waugh, J.S. Scott, M. Cannon

UK, Scotland, North
Scotland-North Cancer Registry (Highlands & Western Isles), Radiotherapy Department, Raigmore Hospital, Inverness IV2 3UJ, Scotland, UK.
Tel: (0463) 34151
M.H. Elia, R. Forrest, M. Palmer

UK, Scotland, North-East
Scotland North-East Cancer Registry, Department of Clinical Oncology, Aberdeen Royal Infirmary, Foresterhill, Aberdeen AB9 2ZB, Scotland, UK.
Tel: (0224) 681818
G. Innes, M. Clark, A.E. Whitter

UK, Scotland, South-East
Scotland South-East Cancer Registry, Liberton Hospital, Lasswade Road, Edinburgh EH16 6UB, Scotland, UK. Tel: (031) 664 4997
G.A. Venters, A.M. McDonald, T. Gilmour, A.M. MacLaren, R.C. Sayers

UK, Scotland, West
Scotland-West Cancer Registry, Greater Glasgow Health Board, Ruchill Hospital, Glasgow G20 9NB, Scotland, UK. Tel: (041) 946 7120
C.R. Gillis, D.J. Hole, D. Lamont, P. Boyle, A. Graham

Yugoslavia, Slovenia
Register raka za SR Slovenijo (Cancer Registry of Slovenia), The Institute of Oncology, Zaloska 2, YU-61105 Ljubljana, Yugoslavia. Tel: (061) 316 490
V. Pompe Kirn, M. Brus, T. Kovacic, N. Robek, A. Valentin-Benedicic, T. Vrevc

OCEANIA

Australian Capital Territory
c/o New South Wales Central Cancer Registry, P.O. Box 380, North Ryde, N.S.W. 2113, Australia.
Tel: (02) 887 5634, Telex: 71675

Joyce Ford, Keithley Bishop, Marylon Coates, Sharon Pettigrew

Australia, New South Wales
New South Wales Central Cancer Registry, P.O. Box 380, North Ryde, N.S.W. 2113, Australia.
Tel: (02) 887 5634, Telex: 71675
Joyce Ford, Keithley Bishop, Marylon Coates, Sharon Pettigrew

Australia, Queensland
Queensland Cancer Registry, Department of Health, G.P.O. Box 48, 147-163 Charlotte Street, Brisbane, Queensland 4001, Australia.
Tel: (07) 227 7187, Telex: AA 42531
I.T. Ring, L. Ward, W. Chant, C. Grodd, T. Paavilainen, S. Webster

South Australia
Central Cancer Registry Unit, South Australian Health Commission, Box 6, Rundle Mall P.O., Adelaide SA 5001, Australia.
Tel: (08) 218 3211, Telex: AA 82925
Anton Bonett, Lesley Milliken, Mary Merdo, Heather Berry, Barbara Hanning, Sue Byrne

Australia, Tasmania
Tasmanian Cancer Registry, GPO Box 709G, Hobart, Tasmania 7001, Australia. Tel: 388698
L.F. Young, K. Jackman

Australia, Victoria
Victorian Cancer Registry, Anti-Cancer Council of Victoria, Keogh House, 1 Rathdowne Street, Carlton South, Victoria 3053, Australia.
Tel: (03) 662 3300, Telex: AA 34158
G. Giles, V. Higgins, M. Dixon, N. Gray

Western Australia
West Australian Cancer Registry Health Department, 60 Beaufort Street, Perth, W. Australia 6000. Tel: (09) 328 0241,
Telex: AA 93111
Mike Hatton, D. Clarke-Hundley, Kaye Garrod, L. Stiring

New Zealand
New Zealand Cancer Registry, National Health Statistics Centre, Ballantrae House, Upper Willis Street, Private Bag 2, Cumberland House Post Office, Wellington, New Zealand. Tel: 844 167, Telex: NZ 3571
F.J. Findlay, J. Fraser, J.A. Auld

USA, Hawaii
Hawaii Tumor Registry, Cancer Center of Hawaii, 1236 Lauhala Street, Room 402, Honolulu, Hawaii 96813, USA. Tel: (808) 521-0054
Laurence N. Kolonel, Marc T. Goodman

Introduction

The *Cancer Incidence in Five Continents* monograph series presents data on the incidence of cancer worldwide. These data are used to generate hypotheses which might explain the enormous differences in the occurrence of many cancers, both between geographical areas of the world and among different ethnic groups within the same area. The work which goes into the collection of reliable statistics on cancer incidence is carried out by population-based cancer registries, and the difficulty of their task is reflected in the unequal geographical representation of worldwide cancer patterns shown here. There are few population-based cancer registries in the continent of Africa, most Latin-American countries and many parts of Asia.

The data which are available show clearly that there are patterns in the occurrence of cancer, within small areas and between different countries. The data from Volume V of *Cancer Incidence in Five Continents,* which was published in 1987 and included standard tabulations of cancer incidence from 137 populations in 36 countries, are depicted here in graphic form. This presentation allows an easier appreciation of the range and pattern of incidence internationally, and highlights the interesting variations for the different cancer sites. Most of the data are for the years 1978-82.

The reliability of the data published in *Cancer Incidence in Five Continents* has been scrutinized very thoroughly. A discussion of the methods used to assess data quality is published in Volume V, and the user of the graphics in the present volume should refer to the publication from which the data are drawn for information on the factors which can produce artefactual differences in the rates. However, given the stringent application of standard editorial criteria to the data published, the rates here can be compared with reasonable confidence.

The user should, however, consult the *Notes on the data* (Table 2) when looking at the figures. The data are coded to the 9th Revision of the International Statistical Classification of Diseases, Injuries and Causes of Death (ICD) (WHO, Manual of the International Statistical Classification of Diseases, Injuries and Causes of Death, Vol. I (Tabular list) and Vol. II (Index), 1975 Revision, Geneva, World Health Organization, 1977), and are presented for all malignant cancers. Abbreviated titles have been used for the graphics, and the user should refer to Table 1 for the full ICD title.

The use of a single classification system is not always interpreted in the same manner, nor is coding always performed in the same way. Differences in practice for individual sites for the majority of terms would almost certainly not have a significant effect on incidence rates, but for the diagnostic statements listed in the *Notes on the data* there could be an effect. The one instance in which there is a marked inflation of the rate for an individual site, the 'Other Endocrine' (ICD-9 194) category, caused by the inclusion of all benign as well as malignant tumours by the Swedish Cancer Registry, has also been footnoted on the histogram.

1

Table 1. – Classification used in graphics – The 9th Revision of the ICD

	Site or type of tumour	Short title used in graphics[a]
140	Malignant neoplasm of lip	Lip
141	Malignant neoplasm of tongue	Tongue
142	Malignant neoplasm of major salivary glands	Salivary gland
143	Malignant neoplasm of gum	
144	Malignant neoplasm of floor of mouth	Mouth
145	Malignant neoplasm of other and unspecified parts of mouth	
146	Malignant neoplasm of oropharynx	Oropharynx
147	Malignant neoplasm of nasopharynx	Nasopharynx
148	Malignant neoplasm of hypopharynx	Hypopharynx
149	Malignant neoplasm of other and ill-defined sites within the lip, oral cavity and pharynx	Pharynx unspec.
150	Malignant neoplasm of oesophagus	Oesophagus
151	Malignant neoplasm of stomach	Stomach
152	Malignant neoplasm of small intestine, including duodenum	Small intestine
153	Malignant neoplasm of colon	Colon
154	Malignant neoplasm of rectum, rectosigmoid junction and anus	Rectum
155	Malignant neoplasm of liver and intrahepatic bile ducts	Liver
156	Malignant neoplasm of gallbladder and extrahepatic bile ducts	Gallbladder etc.
157	Malignant neoplasm of pancreas	Pancreas
158	Malignant neoplasm of retroperitoneum and peritoneum	Peritoneum etc.
159	Malignant neoplasm of other and ill-defined sites within the digestive organs and peritoneum	Primary site uncertain
160	Malignant neoplasm of nasal cavities, middle ear and accessory sinuses	Nose, sinuses etc.
161	Malignant neoplasm of larynx	Larynx
162	Malignant neoplasm of trachea, bronchus and lung	Bronchus, lung
163	Malignant neoplasm of pleura	Pleura
164	Malignant neoplasm of thymus, heart and mediastinum	*Not included separately*
165	Malignant neoplasm of other and ill-defined sites within the respiratory system and intrathoracic organs	Primary site uncertain
170	Malignant neoplasm of bone and articular cartilage	Bone
171	Malignant neoplasm of connective and other soft tissue	Connective tissue
172	Malignant melanoma of skin	Melanoma of skin
173	Other malignant neoplasm of skin	*Not included*
174	Malignant neoplasm of female breast	Breast
175	Malignant neoplasm of male breast	Breast

[a] For specific groupings of sites in the graphics, see pages 3-6

The histograms

The histograms illustrate incidence rates age standardized to the 'world' population for 40 populations in ranking order by site and sex. The populations were chosen to give the widest possible geographical representation. In addition, the highest and lowest rates among *all* the populations included in Volume V of *Cancer Incidence in Five Continents* are given as additional bars at the bottom of each histogram.

Rates based on less than 10 cases have been excluded from the 'lowest' rate given in the final bar. This sometimes results in the 'lowest' rate being higher than the rates for certain of the 40 populations in the histogram, for which rates based on less than 10 cases have been included.

	Site or type of tumour	Short title used in graphics[a]
179	Malignant neoplasm of uterus, part unspecified	Uterus NOS
180	Malignant neoplasm of cervix uteri	Cervix uteri
181	Malignant neoplasm of placenta	Placenta
182	Malignant neoplasm of body of uterus	Corpus uteri
183	Malignant neoplasm of ovary and other uterine adnexa	Ovary etc.
184	Malignant neoplasm of other and unspecified female genital organs	Other female genital
185	Malignant neoplasm of prostate	Prostate
186	Malignant neoplasm of testis	Testis
187	Malignant neoplasm of penis and other male genital organs	Penis etc.
187.1-4	Malignant neoplasm of prepuce, glans penis, body of penis and penis, part unspecified	Penis
188	Malignant neoplasm of bladder	Bladder
189	Malignant neoplasm of kidney and other and unspecified urinary organs	Other urinary
190	Malignant neoplasm of eye	Eye
191	Malignant neoplasm of brain	Brain, nerv. system
192	Malignant neoplasm of other and unspecified parts of nervous system	
193	Malignant neoplasm of thyroid gland	Thyroid
194	Malignant neoplasm of other endocrine glands and related structures	Other endocrine
195	Malignant neoplasm of other and ill-defined sites	Primary site uncertain
196	Secondary and unspecified malignant neoplasm of lymph nodes	Primary site uncertain
197	Secondary malignant neoplasm of respiratory and digestive systems	Primary site uncertain
198	Secondary malignant neoplasm of other specified sites	Primary site uncertain
199	Malignant neoplasm without specification of site	Primary site uncertain
200+202	Lymphosarcoma, reticulosarcoma and other malignant neoplasm of lymphoid and histiocytic tissue	Non-Hodgkin lymphoma
201	Hodgkin's disease	Hodgkin's disease
203	Multiple myeloma and immunoproliferative neoplasms	Multiple myeloma
204	Lymphoid leukaemia	Lymphoid leukaemia
205	Myeloid leukaemia	Myeloid leukaemia
206	Monocytic leukaemia	Monocytic leukaemia
207	Other specified leukaemia	Other leukaemia
208	Leukaemia of unspecified cell type	Leukaemia, cell unspecified

The lowest and highest rates are chosen to the last decimal place. The rates are printed to only one decimal place, so it may appear that, for example, the 'lowest' rate is identical to a rate which appears for a different population in the histogram, as is the case for ICD-9 161 larynx for San Francisco Chinese, and Japan, Miyagi males. In fact the rate for the San Francisco Chinese is very slightly lower than that for Miyagi.

The site groupings used in Volume V have been maintained, i.e. ICD-9 143-145 mouth and ICD-9 191-192 brain and nervous system. In addition it has been decided to group the pharyngeal cancers (ICD-9 146 oropharynx, 148 hypopharynx, and 149 pharynx unspecified), and the non-Hodgkin lymphomas (ICD-9 200 lymphosarcoma, reticulosarcoma and 202 other neoplasms of lymphoid and histiocytic tissue). ICD-9 173 'Other skin' has not been included

Table 2. – Notes on the data

ICD-9 142 includes mixed (salivary) tumours [pleomorphic adenoma of salivary gland]
Israel
Denmark
Hungary, County Vas
Ireland, Southern
Romania, County Cluj
UK, South Thames Region

ICD-9 142 includes mucoepidermoid tumours of the salivary gland
Colombia, Cali
India, Bombay
     Nagpur
     Poona
Israel
Japan, Osaka
Singapore
Denmark
Poland, Warsaw City
Sweden
Australia, Victoria

ICD-9 158 excludes mesothelioma NOS of peritoneum
Brazil, Fortaleza
Colombia, Cali
Hungary, County Szabolcs-Szatmar
     County Vas

ICD-9 158 includes cancers of the peritoneum only (i.e. mesotheliomas)
Finland

ICD-9 158 excludes tumours of retroperitoneum and peritoneum
South Australia

ICD-9 163 excludes mesothelioma NOS of pleura
Brazil, Fortaleza
Colombia, Cali
France, Bas-Rhin
     Doubs
Hungary, County Szabolcs-Szatmar
     County Vas
Sweden

ICD-9 171 includes tumours of retroperitoneum and peritoneum
Finland
South Australia

ICD-9 174 includes intraduct carcinoma of breast
Brazil, Fortaleza
     Pernambuco, Recife
     Porto Alegre
     São Paulo

Colombia, Cali
China, Shanghai
     Tianjin
Hong Kong
Israel
Japan, Osaka
Singapore
German Democratic Republic
Hungary, County Szabolcs-Szatmar
     County Vas
Ireland, Southern
Netherlands, Eindhoven
Poland, Cracow
     Nowy Sacz, Rural Areas
     Warsaw City
Romania, County Cluj
Spain, Navarra
     Zaragoza
UK, Oxford Region
Yugoslavia, Slovenia
New Zealand

ICD-9 180 includes carcinoma in-situ of cervix
Brazil, Pernambuco, Recife
Romania, County Cluj

ICD-9 183 includes ovarian cystadenoma of borderline malignancy
Colombia, Cali
Canada, Alberta
China, Shanghai
India, Bombay
     Nagpur
     Poona
Japan, Osaka
Singapore
Iceland
Netherlands, Eindhoven
Norway
Poland, Cracow
     Nowy Sacz Rural Areas
     Warsaw City
Romania, County Cluj
Australia, Victoria
New Zealand

ICD-9 188 includes unspecified papilloma of bladder
Brazil, Pernambuco, Recife
Colombia, Cali
France, Martinique
India, Bombay
     Nagpur
     Poona

Singapore
Ireland, Southern
Poland, Cracow
      Nowy Sacz Rural Areas
Romania, County Cluj
Switzerland, Zurich

ICD-9 188 includes benign and unspecified papilloma of bladder
Canada, Alberta
USA, California, Los Angeles
Israel
Denmark
Iceland
Italy, Lombardy Region, Varese Province
Norway (includes papilloma of bladder if the
    Bergkvist grading of cellular atypia > 1)
Sweden
Switzerland, Basel
UK, Birmingham & W. Midlands Region
    South Thames Region

ICD-9 191-192 includes benign and/or unspecified neoplasms
Brazil, Fortaleza
      São Paulo
Colombia, Cali
Canada, Alberta
France, Martinique
USA, California, Los Angeles
China, Shanghai
      Tianjin
Israel
Japan, Osaka
Singapore
Denmark
Fed. Rep. of Germany, Saarland
France, Isère
German Democratic Republic
Iceland
Ireland, Southern
Norway
Poland, Cracow
      Nowy Sacz, Rural Areas
      Warsaw City
Romania, County Cluj
Spain, Zaragoza
Sweden
UK, Birmingham & W. Midlands Region
.   South Thames Region

ICD-9 194 includes all benign and malignant tumours
Sweden

because many registries do not collect data on skin cancer. The histogram for all sites of cancer thus includes every malignant category of cancer except for skin cancer.

The 'Primary site uncertain' category gives the incidence of those neoplasms for which a primary site of origin could not be established, i.e. ICD-9 rubrics 195-199, and of other and ill-defined sites within the digestive organs and peritoneum, and within the respiratory system and intrathoracic organs, i.e. rubrics ICD-9 159 and 165.

The colour red is used for males, and blue for females.

Pie diagrams

The pie diagrams give the relative frequencies of the ten top-ranking sites of cancer within each population for which data are published in Volume V. As for the histograms, the site ICD-9 173 'Other skin' has been excluded from the calculations, i.e. it does not appear as one of the top-ranking cancers although it is sufficiently frequent to figure as one of them in many populations, and it is not included in the 'Other cancers' section.

An attempt has been made to label the most frequently occurring sites appropriately: thus bronchus, lung is designated by a pattern of L's and stomach by S's.

The data are arranged by continent – Central and South America, North America, Asia, Europe and Oceania, and alphabetically within continents and countries, as in the list of contributors.

Age-specific rates graphs

The graphs of the age-specific rates show the average annual incidence by sex, selected site and age-group per 100 000 population. The graphs are presented for twenty-four populations from Volume V, chosen for their geographical diversity as for the histograms.

Some of the sites selected have been grouped, as follows:

ICD-9 140-145	Oral cavity (includes lip, tongue, salivary gland and mouth)
ICD-9 146, 148, 149	Pharynx (includes oropharynx, hypopharynx and pharynx unspecified)
ICD-9 153-154	Colon and rectum
ICD-9 191-192	Brain and nervous system
ICD-9 200+202	Non-Hodgkin lymphoma (includes lymphosarcoma and reticulosarcoma, and other malignant neoplasms of lymphoid and histiocytic tissue)
ICD-9 204-208	Leukaemia (includes lymphoid, myeloid, monocytic, other specified and unspecified leukaemia)

Zero rates are represented by gaps in the line of the graph. The red lines are for males and the blue for females.

Part I

Histograms depicting rates of cancer
age-standardized to the 'world' population
by site and sex

140 LIP

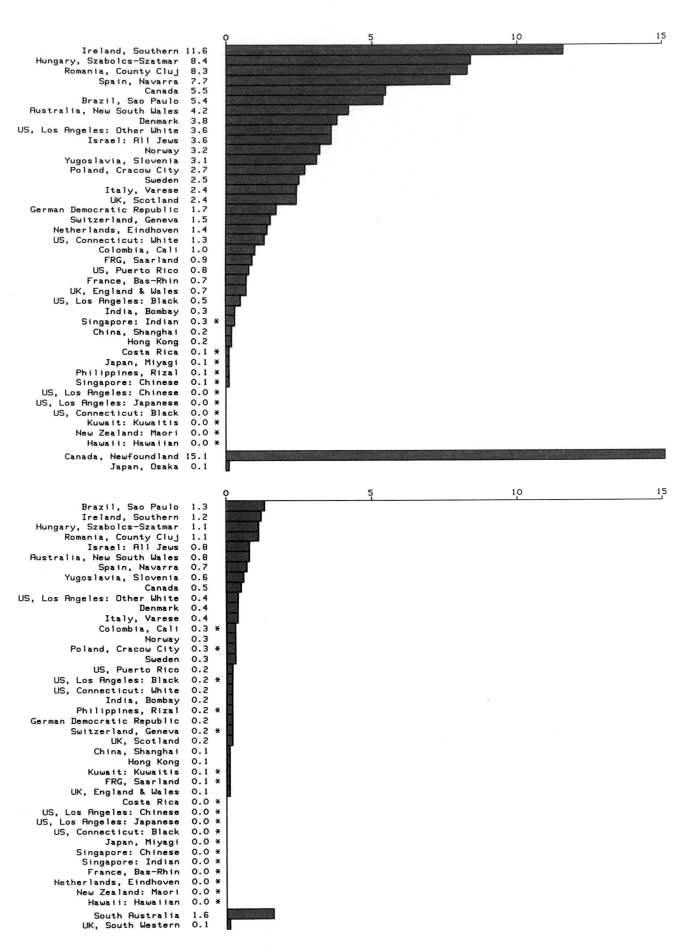

Ireland, Southern 11.6
Hungary, Szabolcs-Szatmar 8.4
Romania, County Cluj 8.3
Spain, Navarra 7.7
Canada 5.5
Brazil, Sao Paulo 5.4
Australia, New South Wales 4.2
Denmark 3.8
US, Los Angeles: Other White 3.6
Israel: All Jews 3.6
Norway 3.2
Yugoslavia, Slovenia 3.1
Poland, Cracow City 2.7
Sweden 2.5
Italy, Varese 2.4
UK, Scotland 2.4
German Democratic Republic 1.7
Switzerland, Geneva 1.5
Netherlands, Eindhoven 1.4
US, Connecticut: White 1.3
Colombia, Cali 1.0
FRG, Saarland 0.9
US, Puerto Rico 0.8
France, Bas-Rhin 0.7
UK, England & Wales 0.7
US, Los Angeles: Black 0.5
India, Bombay 0.3
Singapore: Indian 0.3 *
China, Shanghai 0.2
Hong Kong 0.2
Costa Rica 0.1 *
Japan, Miyagi 0.1 *
Philippines, Rizal 0.1 *
Singapore: Chinese 0.1 *
US, Los Angeles: Chinese 0.0 *
US, Los Angeles: Japanese 0.0 *
US, Connecticut: Black 0.0 *
Kuwait: Kuwaitis 0.0 *
New Zealand: Maori 0.0 *
Hawaii: Hawaiian 0.0 *

Canada, Newfoundland 15.1
Japan, Osaka 0.1

Brazil, Sao Paulo 1.3
Ireland, Southern 1.2
Hungary, Szabolcs-Szatmar 1.1
Romania, County Cluj 1.1
Israel: All Jews 0.8
Australia, New South Wales 0.8
Spain, Navarra 0.7
Yugoslavia, Slovenia 0.6
Canada 0.5
US, Los Angeles: Other White 0.4
Denmark 0.4
Italy, Varese 0.4
Colombia, Cali 0.3 *
Norway 0.3
Poland, Cracow City 0.3 *
Sweden 0.3
US, Puerto Rico 0.2
US, Los Angeles: Black 0.2 *
US, Connecticut: White 0.2
India, Bombay 0.2
Philippines, Rizal 0.2 *
German Democratic Republic 0.2
Switzerland, Geneva 0.2 *
UK, Scotland 0.2
China, Shanghai 0.1
Hong Kong 0.1
Kuwait: Kuwaitis 0.1 *
FRG, Saarland 0.1 *
UK, England & Wales 0.1
Costa Rica 0.0 *
US, Los Angeles: Chinese 0.0 *
US, Los Angeles: Japanese 0.0 *
US, Connecticut: Black 0.0 *
Japan, Miyagi 0.0 *
Singapore: Chinese 0.0 *
Singapore: Indian 0.0 *
France, Bas-Rhin 0.0 *
Netherlands, Eindhoven 0.0 *
New Zealand: Maori 0.0 *
Hawaii: Hawaiian 0.0 *

South Australia 1.6
UK, South Western 0.1

* Rates based on less than 10 cases

8

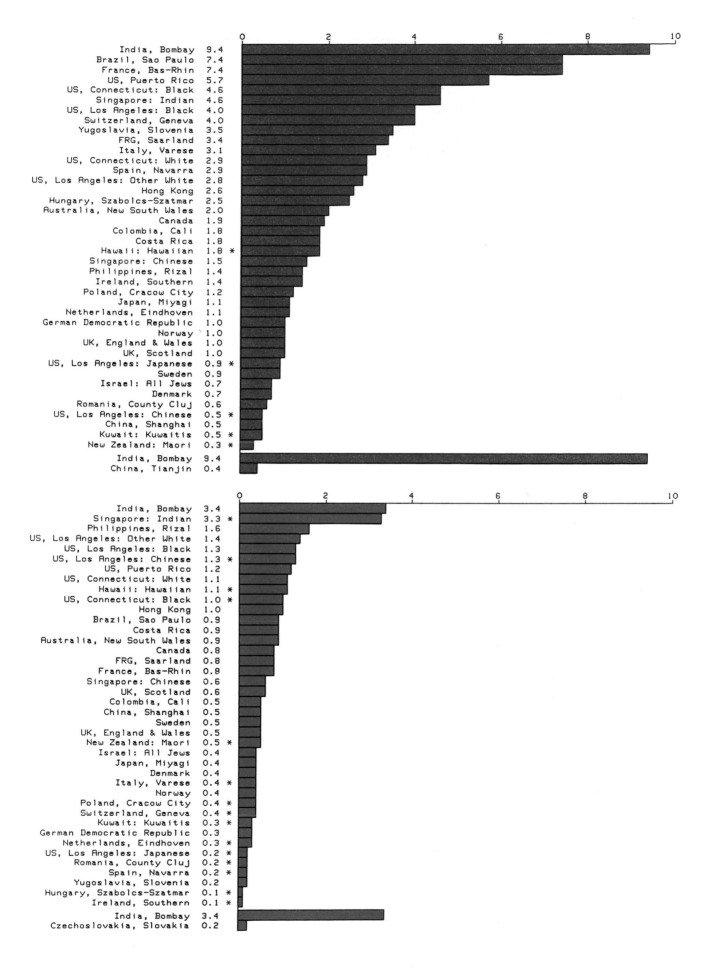

India, Bombay 9.4
Brazil, Sao Paulo 7.4
France, Bas-Rhin 7.4
US, Puerto Rico 5.7
US, Connecticut: Black 4.6
Singapore: Indian 4.6
US, Los Angeles: Black 4.0
Switzerland, Geneva 4.0
Yugoslavia, Slovenia 3.5
FRG, Saarland 3.4
Italy, Varese 3.1
US, Connecticut: White 2.9
Spain, Navarra 2.9
US, Los Angeles: Other White 2.8
Hong Kong 2.6
Hungary, Szabolcs-Szatmar 2.5
Australia, New South Wales 2.0
Canada 1.9
Colombia, Cali 1.8
Costa Rica 1.8
Hawaii: Hawaiian 1.8 *
Singapore: Chinese 1.5
Philippines, Rizal 1.4
Ireland, Southern 1.4
Poland, Cracow City 1.2
Japan, Miyagi 1.1
Netherlands, Eindhoven 1.1
German Democratic Republic 1.0
Norway 1.0
UK, England & Wales 1.0
UK, Scotland 1.0
US, Los Angeles: Japanese 0.9 *
Sweden 0.9
Israel: All Jews 0.7
Denmark 0.7
Romania, County Cluj 0.6
US, Los Angeles: Chinese 0.5 *
China, Shanghai 0.5
Kuwait: Kuwaitis 0.5 *
New Zealand: Maori 0.3 *

India, Bombay 9.4
China, Tianjin 0.4

India, Bombay 3.4
Singapore: Indian 3.3 *
Philippines, Rizal 1.6
US, Los Angeles: Other White 1.4
US, Los Angeles: Black 1.3
US, Los Angeles: Chinese 1.3 *
US, Puerto Rico 1.2
US, Connecticut: White 1.1
Hawaii: Hawaiian 1.1 *
US, Connecticut: Black 1.0 *
Hong Kong 1.0
Brazil, Sao Paulo 0.9
Costa Rica 0.9
Australia, New South Wales 0.9
Canada 0.8
FRG, Saarland 0.8
France, Bas-Rhin 0.8
Singapore: Chinese 0.6
UK, Scotland 0.6
Colombia, Cali 0.5
China, Shanghai 0.5
Sweden 0.5
UK, England & Wales 0.5
New Zealand: Maori 0.5 *
Israel: All Jews 0.4
Japan, Miyagi 0.4
Denmark 0.4
Italy, Varese 0.4 *
Norway 0.4
Poland, Cracow City 0.4 *
Switzerland, Geneva 0.4 *
Kuwait: Kuwaitis 0.3 *
German Democratic Republic 0.3
Netherlands, Eindhoven 0.3 *
US, Los Angeles: Japanese 0.2 *
Romania, County Cluj 0.2 *
Spain, Navarra 0.2 *
Yugoslavia, Slovenia 0.2
Hungary, Szabolcs-Szatmar 0.1 *
Ireland, Southern 0.1 *

India, Bombay 3.4
Czechoslovakia, Slovakia 0.2

* Rates based on less than 10 cases

142 SALIVARY GLAND

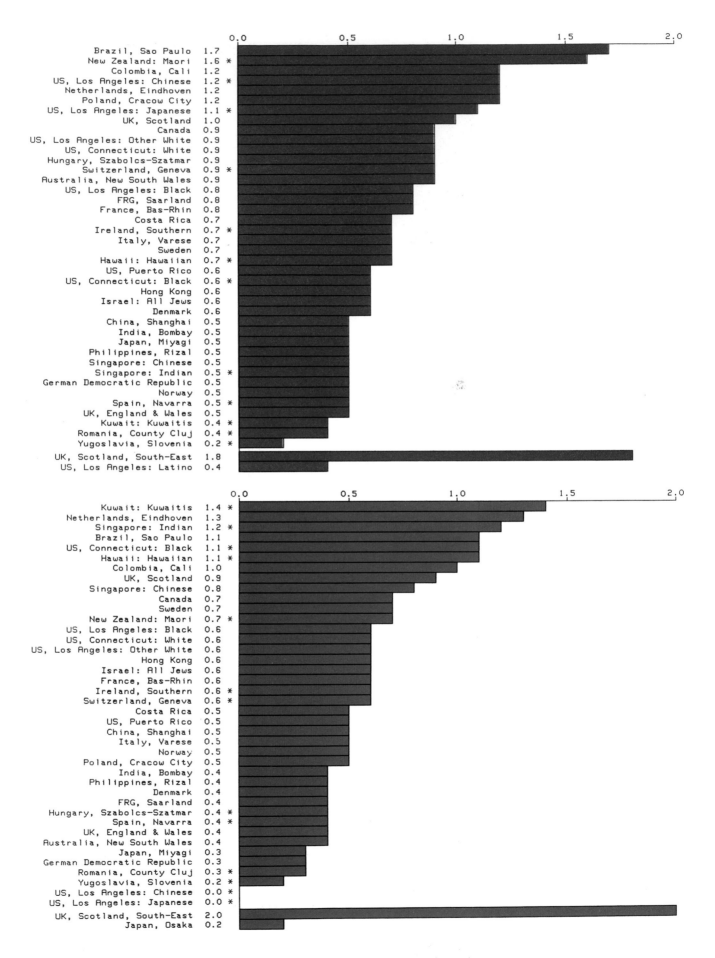

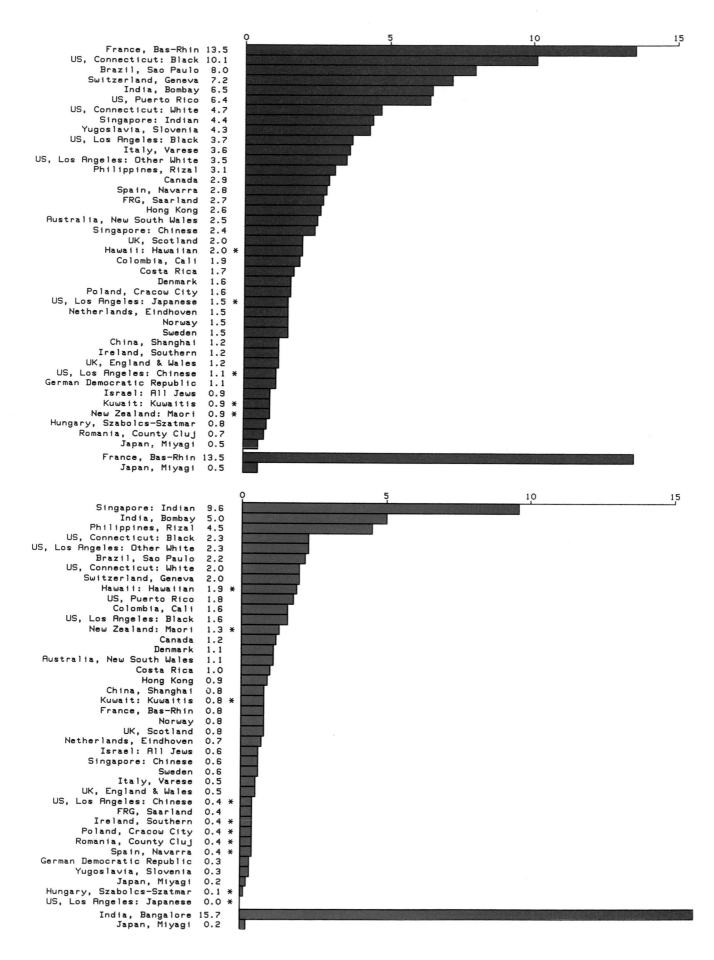

* Rates based on less than 10 cases

147 NASOPHARYNX

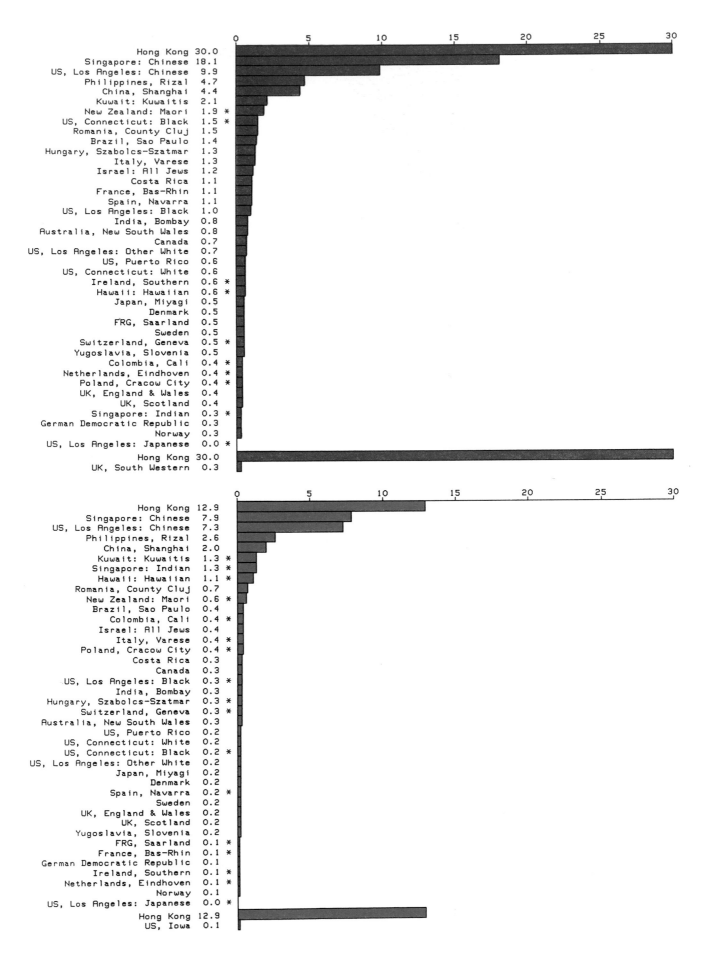

* Rates based on less than 10 cases

146, 148, 149 OROPHARYNX, HYPOPHARYNX AND PHARYNX UNSPEC.

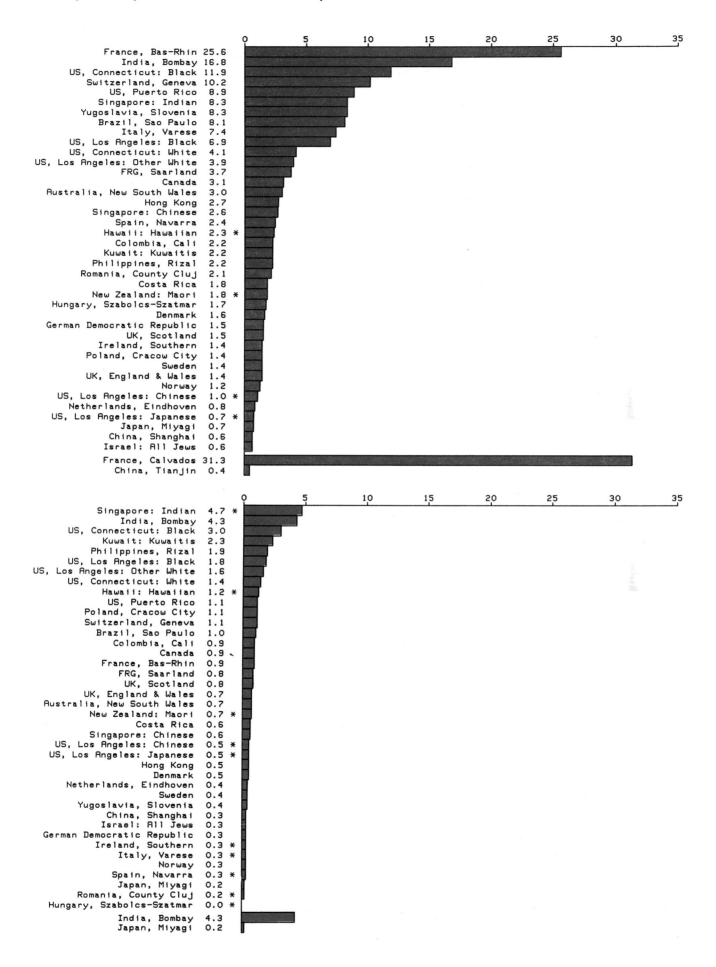

France, Bas-Rhin	25.6
India, Bombay	16.8
US, Connecticut: Black	11.9
Switzerland, Geneva	10.2
US, Puerto Rico	8.9
Singapore: Indian	8.3
Yugoslavia, Slovenia	8.3
Brazil, Sao Paulo	8.1
Italy, Varese	7.4
US, Los Angeles: Black	6.9
US, Connecticut: White	4.1
US, Los Angeles: Other White	3.9
FRG, Saarland	3.7
Canada	3.1
Australia, New South Wales	3.0
Hong Kong	2.7
Singapore: Chinese	2.6
Spain, Navarra	2.4
Hawaii: Hawaiian	2.3 *
Colombia, Cali	2.2
Kuwait: Kuwaitis	2.2
Philippines, Rizal	2.2
Romania, County Cluj	2.1
Costa Rica	1.8
New Zealand: Maori	1.8 *
Hungary, Szabolcs-Szatmar	1.7
Denmark	1.6
German Democratic Republic	1.5
UK, Scotland	1.5
Ireland, Southern	1.4
Poland, Cracow City	1.4
Sweden	1.4
UK, England & Wales	1.4
Norway	1.2
US, Los Angeles: Chinese	1.0 *
Netherlands, Eindhoven	0.8
US, Los Angeles: Japanese	0.7 *
Japan, Miyagi	0.7
China, Shanghai	0.6
Israel: All Jews	0.6
France, Calvados	31.3
China, Tianjin	0.4

Singapore: Indian	4.7 *
India, Bombay	4.3
US, Connecticut: Black	3.0
Kuwait: Kuwaitis	2.3
Philippines, Rizal	1.9
US, Los Angeles: Black	1.8
US, Los Angeles: Other White	1.6
US, Connecticut: White	1.4
Hawaii: Hawaiian	1.2 *
US, Puerto Rico	1.1
Poland, Cracow City	1.1
Switzerland, Geneva	1.1
Brazil, Sao Paulo	1.0
Colombia, Cali	0.9
Canada	0.9
France, Bas-Rhin	0.9
FRG, Saarland	0.8
UK, Scotland	0.8
UK, England & Wales	0.7
Australia, New South Wales	0.7
New Zealand: Maori	0.7 *
Costa Rica	0.6
Singapore: Chinese	0.6
US, Los Angeles: Chinese	0.5 *
US, Los Angeles: Japanese	0.5 *
Hong Kong	0.5
Denmark	0.5
Netherlands, Eindhoven	0.4
Sweden	0.4
Yugoslavia, Slovenia	0.4
China, Shanghai	0.3
Israel: All Jews	0.3
German Democratic Republic	0.3
Ireland, Southern	0.3 *
Italy, Varese	0.3 *
Norway	0.3
Spain, Navarra	0.3 *
Japan, Miyagi	0.2
Romania, County Cluj	0.2 *
Hungary, Szabolcs-Szatmar	0.0 *
India, Bombay	4.3
Japan, Miyagi	0.2

* Rates based on less than 10 cases

13

150 OESOPHAGUS

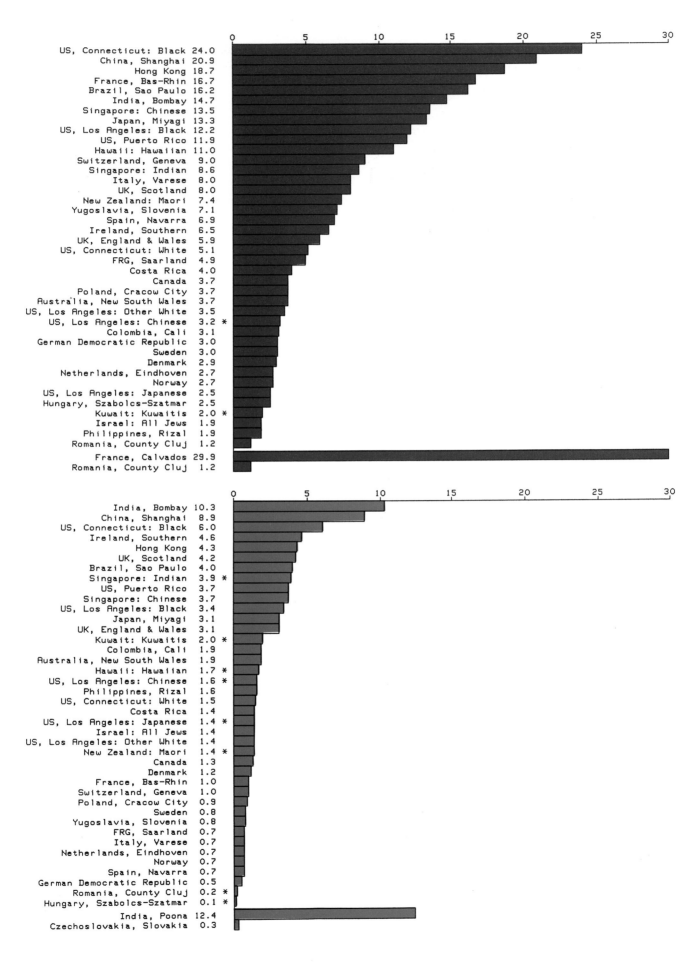

US, Connecticut: Black	24.0
China, Shanghai	20.9
Hong Kong	18.7
France, Bas-Rhin	16.7
Brazil, Sao Paulo	16.2
India, Bombay	14.7
Singapore: Chinese	13.5
Japan, Miyagi	13.3
US, Los Angeles: Black	12.2
US, Puerto Rico	11.9
Hawaii: Hawaiian	11.0
Switzerland, Geneva	9.0
Singapore: Indian	8.6
Italy, Varese	8.0
UK, Scotland	8.0
New Zealand: Maori	7.4
Yugoslavia, Slovenia	7.1
Spain, Navarra	6.9
Ireland, Southern	6.5
UK, England & Wales	5.9
US, Connecticut: White	5.1
FRG, Saarland	4.9
Costa Rica	4.0
Canada	3.7
Poland, Cracow City	3.7
Australia, New South Wales	3.7
US, Los Angeles: Other White	3.5
US, Los Angeles: Chinese	3.2 *
Colombia, Cali	3.1
German Democratic Republic	3.0
Sweden	3.0
Denmark	2.9
Netherlands, Eindhoven	2.7
Norway	2.7
US, Los Angeles: Japanese	2.5
Hungary, Szabolcs-Szatmar	2.5
Kuwait: Kuwaitis	2.0 *
Israel: All Jews	1.9
Philippines, Rizal	1.9
Romania, County Cluj	1.2
France, Calvados	29.9
Romania, County Cluj	1.2

India, Bombay	10.3
China, Shanghai	8.9
US, Connecticut: Black	6.0
Ireland, Southern	4.6
Hong Kong	4.3
UK, Scotland	4.2
Brazil, Sao Paulo	4.0
Singapore: Indian	3.9 *
US, Puerto Rico	3.7
Singapore: Chinese	3.7
US, Los Angeles: Black	3.4
Japan, Miyagi	3.1
UK, England & Wales	3.1
Kuwait: Kuwaitis	2.0 *
Colombia, Cali	1.9
Australia, New South Wales	1.9
Hawaii: Hawaiian	1.7 *
US, Los Angeles: Chinese	1.6 *
Philippines, Rizal	1.6
US, Connecticut: White	1.5
Costa Rica	1.4
US, Los Angeles: Japanese	1.4 *
Israel: All Jews	1.4
US, Los Angeles: Other White	1.4
New Zealand: Maori	1.4 *
Canada	1.3
Denmark	1.2
France, Bas-Rhin	1.0
Switzerland, Geneva	1.0
Poland, Cracow City	0.9
Sweden	0.8
Yugoslavia, Slovenia	0.8
FRG, Saarland	0.7
Italy, Varese	0.7
Netherlands, Eindhoven	0.7
Norway	0.7
Spain, Navarra	0.7
German Democratic Republic	0.5
Romania, County Cluj	0.2 *
Hungary, Szabolcs-Szatmar	0.1 *
India, Poona	12.4
Czechoslovakia, Slovakia	0.3

* Rates based on less than 10 cases

14

151 STOMACH

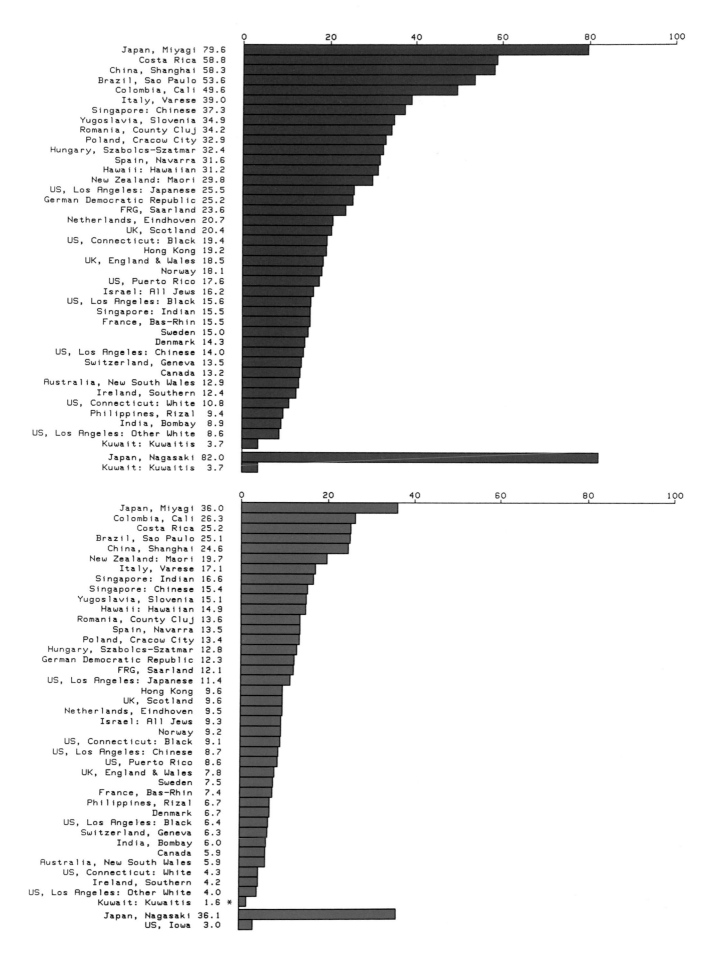

152 SMALL INTESTINE

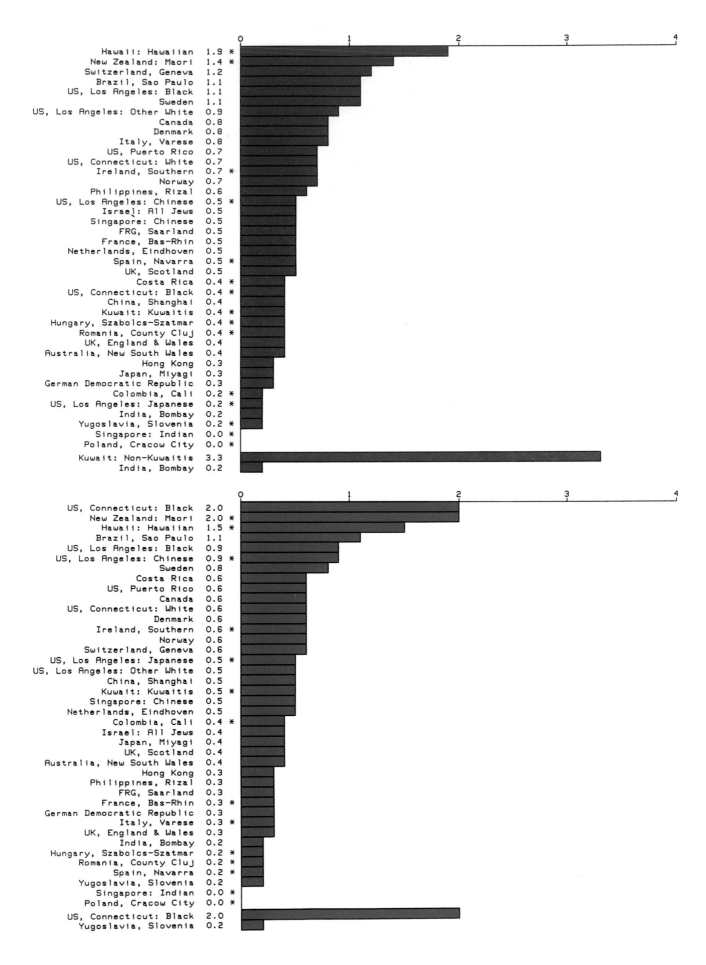

Hawaii: Hawaiian	1.9 *
New Zealand: Maori	1.4 *
Switzerland, Geneva	1.2
Brazil, Sao Paulo	1.1
US, Los Angeles: Black	1.1
Sweden	1.1
US, Los Angeles: Other White	0.9
Canada	0.8
Denmark	0.8
Italy, Varese	0.8
US, Puerto Rico	0.7
US, Connecticut: White	0.7
Ireland, Southern	0.7 *
Norway	0.7
Philippines, Rizal	0.6
US, Los Angeles: Chinese	0.5 *
Israel: All Jews	0.5
Singapore: Chinese	0.5
FRG, Saarland	0.5
France, Bas-Rhin	0.5
Netherlands, Eindhoven	0.5
Spain, Navarra	0.5 *
UK, Scotland	0.5
Costa Rica	0.4 *
US, Connecticut: Black	0.4 *
China, Shanghai	0.4
Kuwait: Kuwaitis	0.4 *
Hungary, Szabolcs-Szatmar	0.4 *
Romania, County Cluj	0.4 *
UK, England & Wales	0.4
Australia, New South Wales	0.4
Hong Kong	0.3
Japan, Miyagi	0.3
German Democratic Republic	0.3
Colombia, Cali	0.2 *
US, Los Angeles: Japanese	0.2 *
India, Bombay	0.2
Yugoslavia, Slovenia	0.2 *
Singapore: Indian	0.0 *
Poland, Cracow City	0.0 *
Kuwait: Non-Kuwaitis	3.3
India, Bombay	0.2

US, Connecticut: Black	2.0
New Zealand: Maori	2.0 *
Hawaii: Hawaiian	1.5 *
Brazil, Sao Paulo	1.1
US, Los Angeles: Black	0.9
US, Los Angeles: Chinese	0.9 *
Sweden	0.8
Costa Rica	0.6
US, Puerto Rico	0.6
Canada	0.6
US, Connecticut: White	0.6
Denmark	0.6
Ireland, Southern	0.6 *
Norway	0.6
Switzerland, Geneva	0.6
US, Los Angeles: Japanese	0.5 *
US, Los Angeles: Other White	0.5
China, Shanghai	0.5
Kuwait: Kuwaitis	0.5 *
Singapore: Chinese	0.5
Netherlands, Eindhoven	0.5
Colombia, Cali	0.4 *
Israel: All Jews	0.4
Japan, Miyagi	0.4
UK, Scotland	0.4
Australia, New South Wales	0.4
Hong Kong	0.3
Philippines, Rizal	0.3
FRG, Saarland	0.3
France, Bas-Rhin	0.3 *
German Democratic Republic	0.3
Italy, Varese	0.3 *
UK, England & Wales	0.3
India, Bombay	0.2
Hungary, Szabolcs-Szatmar	0.2 *
Romania, County Cluj	0.2 *
Spain, Navarra	0.2 *
Yugoslavia, Slovenia	0.2
Singapore: Indian	0.0 *
Poland, Cracow City	0.0
US, Connecticut: Black	2.0
Yugoslavia, Slovenia	0.2

* Rates based on less than 10 cases

16

153 COLON

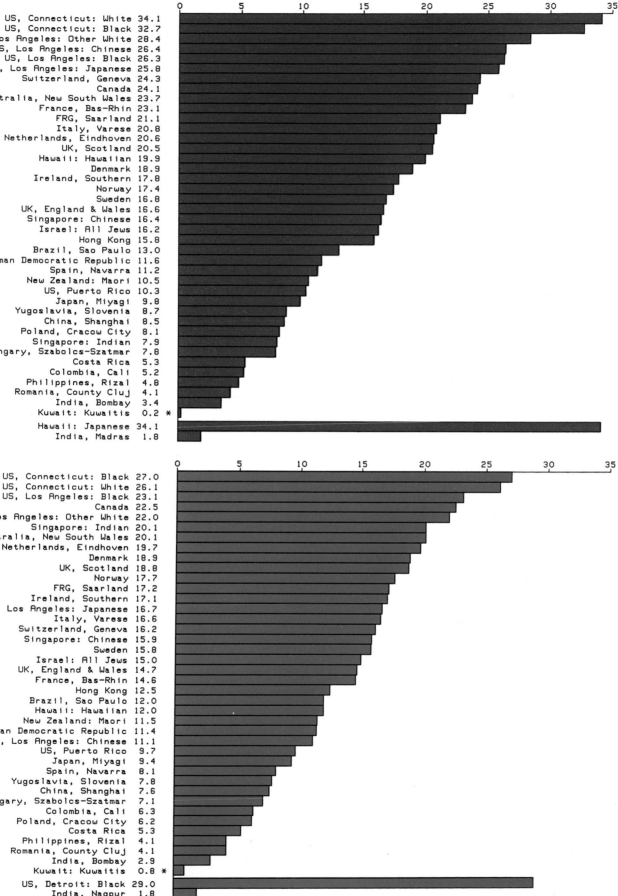

US, Connecticut: White 34.1
US, Connecticut: Black 32.7
US, Los Angeles: Other White 28.4
US, Los Angeles: Chinese 26.4
US, Los Angeles: Black 26.3
US, Los Angeles: Japanese 25.8
Switzerland, Geneva 24.3
Canada 24.1
Australia, New South Wales 23.7
France, Bas-Rhin 23.1
FRG, Saarland 21.1
Italy, Varese 20.8
Netherlands, Eindhoven 20.6
UK, Scotland 20.5
Hawaii: Hawaiian 19.9
Denmark 18.9
Ireland, Southern 17.8
Norway 17.4
Sweden 16.8
UK, England & Wales 16.6
Singapore: Chinese 16.4
Israel: All Jews 16.2
Hong Kong 15.8
Brazil, Sao Paulo 13.0
German Democratic Republic 11.6
Spain, Navarra 11.2
New Zealand: Maori 10.5
US, Puerto Rico 10.3
Japan, Miyagi 9.8
Yugoslavia, Slovenia 8.7
China, Shanghai 8.5
Poland, Cracow City 8.1
Singapore: Indian 7.9
Hungary, Szabolcs-Szatmar 7.8
Costa Rica 5.3
Colombia, Cali 5.2
Philippines, Rizal 4.8
Romania, County Cluj 4.1
India, Bombay 3.4
Kuwait: Kuwaitis 0.2 *

Hawaii: Japanese 34.1
India, Madras 1.8

US, Connecticut: Black 27.0
US, Connecticut: White 26.1
US, Los Angeles: Black 23.1
Canada 22.5
US, Los Angeles: Other White 22.0
Singapore: Indian 20.1
Australia, New South Wales 20.1
Netherlands, Eindhoven 19.7
Denmark 18.9
UK, Scotland 18.8
Norway 17.7
FRG, Saarland 17.2
Ireland, Southern 17.1
US, Los Angeles: Japanese 16.7
Italy, Varese 16.6
Switzerland, Geneva 16.2
Singapore: Chinese 15.9
Sweden 15.8
Israel: All Jews 15.0
UK, England & Wales 14.7
France, Bas-Rhin 14.6
Hong Kong 12.5
Brazil, Sao Paulo 12.0
Hawaii: Hawaiian 12.0
New Zealand: Maori 11.5
German Democratic Republic 11.4
US, Los Angeles: Chinese 11.1
US, Puerto Rico 9.7
Japan, Miyagi 9.4
Spain, Navarra 8.1
Yugoslavia, Slovenia 7.8
China, Shanghai 7.6
Hungary, Szabolcs-Szatmar 7.1
Colombia, Cali 6.3
Poland, Cracow City 6.2
Costa Rica 5.3
Philippines, Rizal 4.1
Romania, County Cluj 4.1
India, Bombay 2.9
Kuwait: Kuwaitis 0.8 *

US, Detroit: Black 29.0
India, Nagpur 1.8

* Rates based on less than 10 cases

154 RECTUM

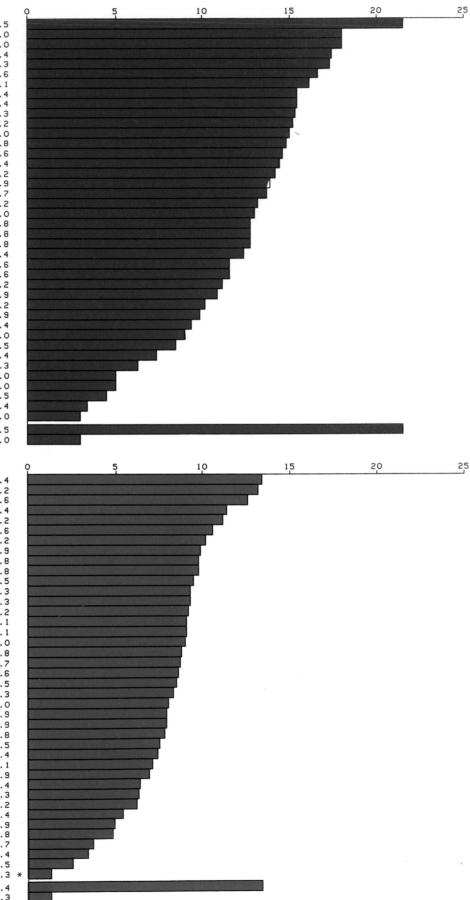

FRG, Saarland 21.5
US, Connecticut: White 18.0
France, Bas-Rhin 18.0
Denmark 17.4
Italy, Varese 17.3
Israel: All Jews 16.6
Hawaii: Hawaiian 16.1
US, Los Angeles: Chinese 15.4
Australia, New South Wales 15.4
Canada 15.3
US, Los Angeles: Japanese 15.2
Netherlands, Eindhoven 15.0
Norway 14.8
Singapore: Chinese 14.6
Yugoslavia, Slovenia 14.4
US, Los Angeles: Other White 14.2
German Democratic Republic 13.9
UK, England & Wales 13.7
UK, Scotland 13.2
Ireland, Southern 13.0
US, Los Angeles: Black 12.8
US, Connecticut: Black 12.8
Switzerland, Geneva 12.8
Hong Kong 12.4
Sweden 11.6
New Zealand: Maori 11.6
Spain, Navarra 11.2
Hungary, Szabolcs-Szatmar 10.9
Poland, Cracow City 10.2
Japan, Miyagi 9.9
China, Shanghai 9.4
Brazil, Sao Paulo 9.0
Romania, County Cluj 8.5
US, Puerto Rico 7.4
Singapore: Indian 6.3
Costa Rica 5.0
Philippines, Rizal 5.0
India, Bombay 4.5
Colombia, Cali 3.4
Kuwait: Kuwaitis 3.0

FRG, Saarland 21.5
Kuwait: Kuwaitis 3.0

Israel: All Jews 13.4
FRG, Saarland 13.2
US, Los Angeles: Japanese 12.6
US, Connecticut: White 11.4
Denmark 11.2
Singapore: Chinese 10.6
Norway 10.2
German Democratic Republic 9.9
Canada 9.8
Switzerland, Geneva 9.8
US, Los Angeles: Other White 9.5
Singapore: Indian 9.3
Australia, New South Wales 9.3
Hong Kong 9.2
Brazil, Sao Paulo 9.1
Netherlands, Eindhoven 9.1
Italy, Varese 9.0
US, Los Angeles: Chinese 8.8
Yugoslavia, Slovenia 8.7
Ireland, Southern 8.6
France, Bas-Rhin 8.5
UK, Scotland 8.3
US, Los Angeles: Black 8.0
US, Connecticut: Black 7.9
UK, England & Wales 7.9
Sweden 7.8
Spain, Navarra 7.5
Japan, Miyagi 7.4
China, Shanghai 7.1
Hawaii: Hawaiian 6.9
Romania, County Cluj 6.4
Hungary, Szabolcs-Szatmar 6.3
Poland, Cracow City 6.2
US, Puerto Rico 5.4
Costa Rica 4.9
New Zealand: Maori 4.8
Colombia, Cali 3.7
Philippines, Rizal 3.4
India, Bombay 2.5
Kuwait: Kuwaitis 1.3 *

Israel: All Jews 13.4
India, Madras 1.3

* Rates based on less than 10 cases

155 LIVER

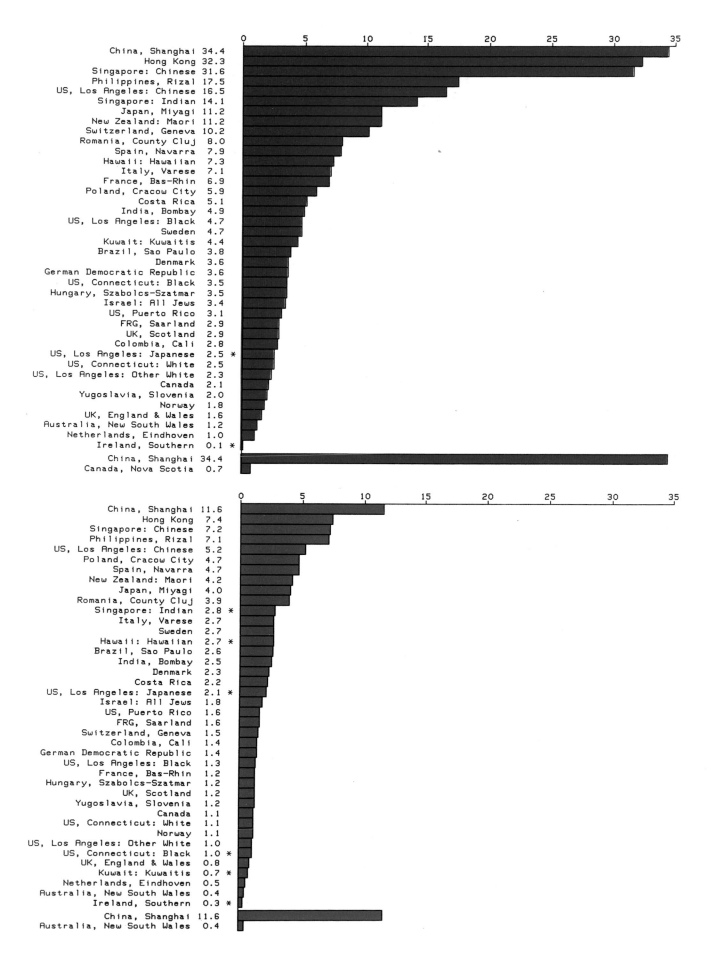

China, Shanghai 34.4
Hong Kong 32.3
Singapore: Chinese 31.6
Philippines, Rizal 17.5
US, Los Angeles: Chinese 16.5
Singapore: Indian 14.1
Japan, Miyagi 11.2
New Zealand: Maori 11.2
Switzerland, Geneva 10.2
Romania, County Cluj 8.0
Spain, Navarra 7.9
Hawaii: Hawaiian 7.3
Italy, Varese 7.1
France, Bas-Rhin 6.9
Poland, Cracow City 5.9
Costa Rica 5.1
India, Bombay 4.9
US, Los Angeles: Black 4.7
Sweden 4.7
Kuwait: Kuwaitis 4.4
Brazil, Sao Paulo 3.8
Denmark 3.6
German Democratic Republic 3.6
US, Connecticut: Black 3.5
Hungary, Szabolcs-Szatmar 3.5
Israel: All Jews 3.4
US, Puerto Rico 3.1
FRG, Saarland 2.9
UK, Scotland 2.9
Colombia, Cali 2.8
US, Los Angeles: Japanese 2.5 *
US, Connecticut: White 2.5
US, Los Angeles: Other White 2.3
Canada 2.1
Yugoslavia, Slovenia 2.0
Norway 1.8
UK, England & Wales 1.6
Australia, New South Wales 1.2
Netherlands, Eindhoven 1.0
Ireland, Southern 0.1 *
China, Shanghai 34.4
Canada, Nova Scotia 0.7

China, Shanghai 11.6
Hong Kong 7.4
Singapore: Chinese 7.2
Philippines, Rizal 7.1
US, Los Angeles: Chinese 5.2
Poland, Cracow City 4.7
Spain, Navarra 4.7
New Zealand: Maori 4.2
Japan, Miyagi 4.0
Romania, County Cluj 3.9
Singapore: Indian 2.8 *
Italy, Varese 2.7
Sweden 2.7
Hawaii: Hawaiian 2.7 *
Brazil, Sao Paulo 2.6
India, Bombay 2.5
Denmark 2.3
Costa Rica 2.2
US, Los Angeles: Japanese 2.1 *
Israel: All Jews 1.8
US, Puerto Rico 1.6
FRG, Saarland 1.6
Switzerland, Geneva 1.5
Colombia, Cali 1.4
German Democratic Republic 1.4
US, Los Angeles: Black 1.3
France, Bas-Rhin 1.2
Hungary, Szabolcs-Szatmar 1.2
UK, Scotland 1.2
Yugoslavia, Slovenia 1.2
Canada 1.1
US, Connecticut: White 1.1
Norway 1.1
US, Los Angeles: Other White 1.0
US, Connecticut: Black 1.0 *
UK, England & Wales 0.8
Kuwait: Kuwaitis 0.7 *
Netherlands, Eindhoven 0.5
Australia, New South Wales 0.4
Ireland, Southern 0.3 *
China, Shanghai 11.6
Australia, New South Wales 0.4

* Rates based on less than 10 cases

19

156 GALLBLADDER ETC.

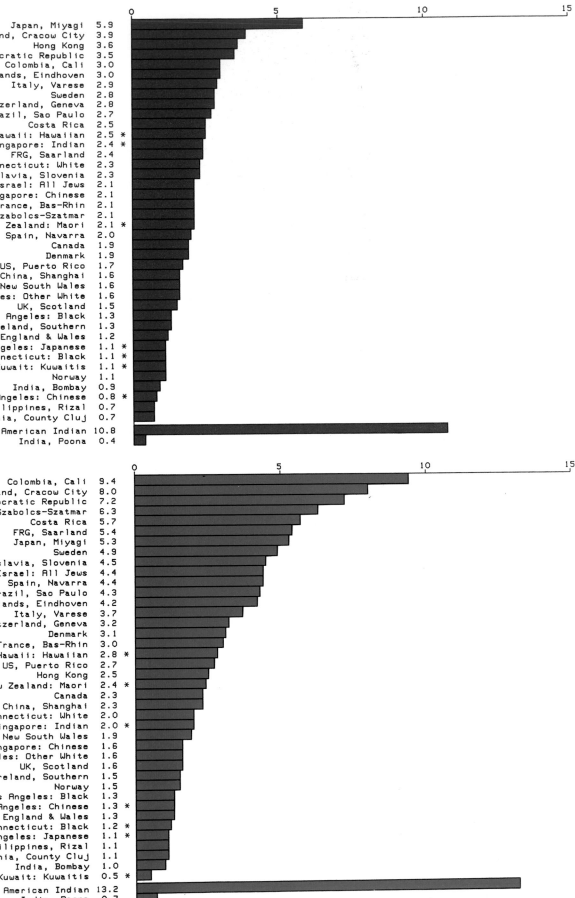

Japan, Miyagi	5.9
Poland, Cracow City	3.9
Hong Kong	3.6
German Democratic Republic	3.5
Colombia, Cali	3.0
Netherlands, Eindhoven	3.0
Italy, Varese	2.9
Sweden	2.8
Switzerland, Geneva	2.8
Brazil, Sao Paulo	2.7
Costa Rica	2.5
Hawaii: Hawaiian	2.5 *
Singapore: Indian	2.4 *
FRG, Saarland	2.4
US, Connecticut: White	2.3
Yugoslavia, Slovenia	2.3
Israel: All Jews	2.1
Singapore: Chinese	2.1
France, Bas-Rhin	2.1
Hungary, Szabolcs-Szatmar	2.1
New Zealand: Maori	2.1 *
Spain, Navarra	2.0
Canada	1.9
Denmark	1.9
US, Puerto Rico	1.7
China, Shanghai	1.6
Australia, New South Wales	1.6
US, Los Angeles: Other White	1.6
UK, Scotland	1.5
US, Los Angeles: Black	1.3
Ireland, Southern	1.3
UK, England & Wales	1.2
US, Los Angeles: Japanese	1.1 *
US, Connecticut: Black	1.1 *
Kuwait: Kuwaitis	1.1 *
Norway	1.1
India, Bombay	0.9
US, Los Angeles: Chinese	0.8 *
Philippines, Rizal	0.7
Romania, County Cluj	0.7
US, New Mexico: American Indian	10.8
India, Poona	0.4

Colombia, Cali	9.4
Poland, Cracow City	8.0
German Democratic Republic	7.2
Hungary, Szabolcs-Szatmar	6.3
Costa Rica	5.7
FRG, Saarland	5.4
Japan, Miyagi	5.3
Sweden	4.9
Yugoslavia, Slovenia	4.5
Israel: All Jews	4.4
Spain, Navarra	4.4
Brazil, Sao Paulo	4.3
Netherlands, Eindhoven	4.2
Italy, Varese	3.7
Switzerland, Geneva	3.2
Denmark	3.1
France, Bas-Rhin	3.0
Hawaii: Hawaiian	2.8 *
US, Puerto Rico	2.7
Hong Kong	2.5
New Zealand: Maori	2.4 *
Canada	2.3
China, Shanghai	2.3
US, Connecticut: White	2.0
Singapore: Indian	2.0 *
Australia, New South Wales	1.9
Singapore: Chinese	1.6
US, Los Angeles: Other White	1.6
UK, Scotland	1.6
Ireland, Southern	1.5
Norway	1.5
US, Los Angeles: Black	1.3
US, Los Angeles: Chinese	1.3 *
UK, England & Wales	1.3
US, Connecticut: Black	1.2 *
US, Los Angeles: Japanese	1.1 *
Philippines, Rizal	1.1
Romania, County Cluj	1.1
India, Bombay	1.0
Kuwait: Kuwaitis	0.5 *
US, New Mexico: American Indian	13.2
India, Poona	0.7

* Rates based on less than 10 cases

157 PANCREAS

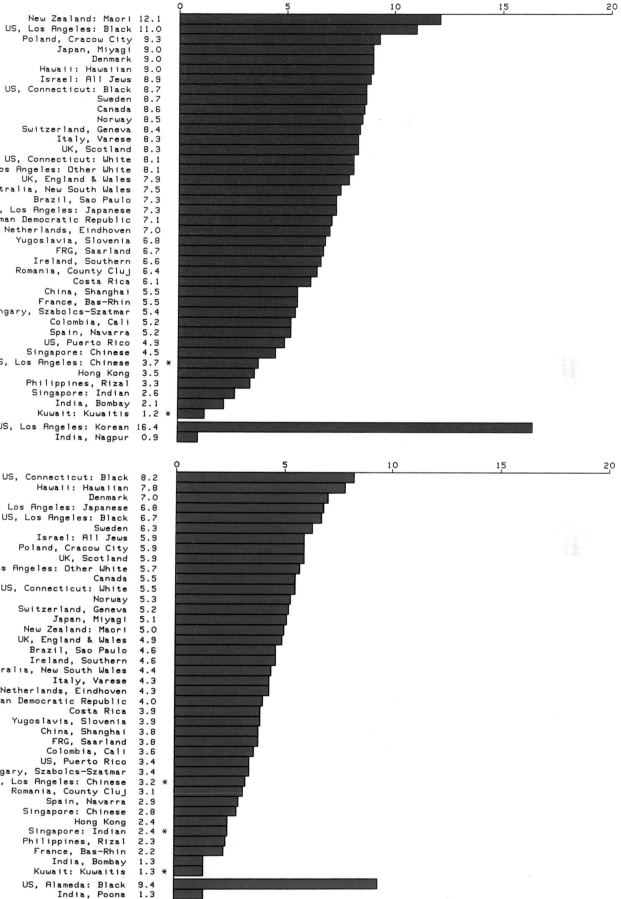

New Zealand: Maori	12.1
US, Los Angeles: Black	11.0
Poland, Cracow City	9.3
Japan, Miyagi	9.0
Denmark	9.0
Hawaii: Hawaiian	9.0
Israel: All Jews	8.9
US, Connecticut: Black	8.7
Sweden	8.7
Canada	8.6
Norway	8.5
Switzerland, Geneva	8.4
Italy, Varese	8.3
UK, Scotland	8.3
US, Connecticut: White	8.1
US, Los Angeles: Other White	8.1
UK, England & Wales	7.9
Australia, New South Wales	7.5
Brazil, Sao Paulo	7.3
US, Los Angeles: Japanese	7.3
German Democratic Republic	7.1
Netherlands, Eindhoven	7.0
Yugoslavia, Slovenia	6.8
FRG, Saarland	6.7
Ireland, Southern	6.6
Romania, County Cluj	6.4
Costa Rica	6.1
China, Shanghai	5.5
France, Bas-Rhin	5.5
Hungary, Szabolcs-Szatmar	5.4
Colombia, Cali	5.2
Spain, Navarra	5.2
US, Puerto Rico	4.9
Singapore: Chinese	4.5
US, Los Angeles: Chinese	3.7 *
Hong Kong	3.5
Philippines, Rizal	3.3
Singapore: Indian	2.6
India, Bombay	2.1
Kuwait: Kuwaitis	1.2 *
US, Los Angeles: Korean	16.4
India, Nagpur	0.9

US, Connecticut: Black	8.2
Hawaii: Hawaiian	7.8
Denmark	7.0
US, Los Angeles: Japanese	6.8
US, Los Angeles: Black	6.7
Sweden	6.3
Israel: All Jews	5.9
Poland, Cracow City	5.9
UK, Scotland	5.9
US, Los Angeles: Other White	5.7
Canada	5.5
US, Connecticut: White	5.5
Norway	5.3
Switzerland, Geneva	5.2
Japan, Miyagi	5.1
New Zealand: Maori	5.0
UK, England & Wales	4.9
Brazil, Sao Paulo	4.6
Ireland, Southern	4.6
Australia, New South Wales	4.4
Italy, Varese	4.3
Netherlands, Eindhoven	4.3
German Democratic Republic	4.0
Costa Rica	3.9
Yugoslavia, Slovenia	3.9
China, Shanghai	3.8
FRG, Saarland	3.8
Colombia, Cali	3.6
US, Puerto Rico	3.4
Hungary, Szabolcs-Szatmar	3.4
US, Los Angeles: Chinese	3.2 *
Romania, County Cluj	3.1
Spain, Navarra	2.9
Singapore: Chinese	2.8
Hong Kong	2.4
Singapore: Indian	2.4 *
Philippines, Rizal	2.3
France, Bas-Rhin	2.2
India, Bombay	1.3
Kuwait: Kuwaitis	1.3 *
US, Alameda: Black	9.4
India, Poona	1.3

* Rates based on less than 10 cases

21

158 PERITONEUM ETC.

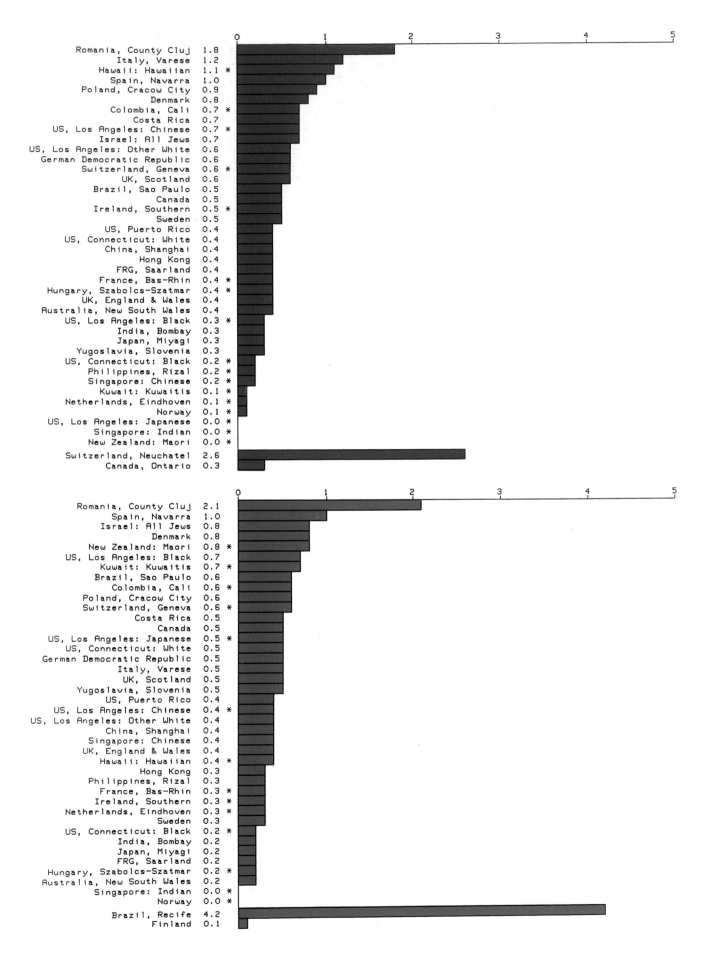

160 NOSE, SINUSES ETC.

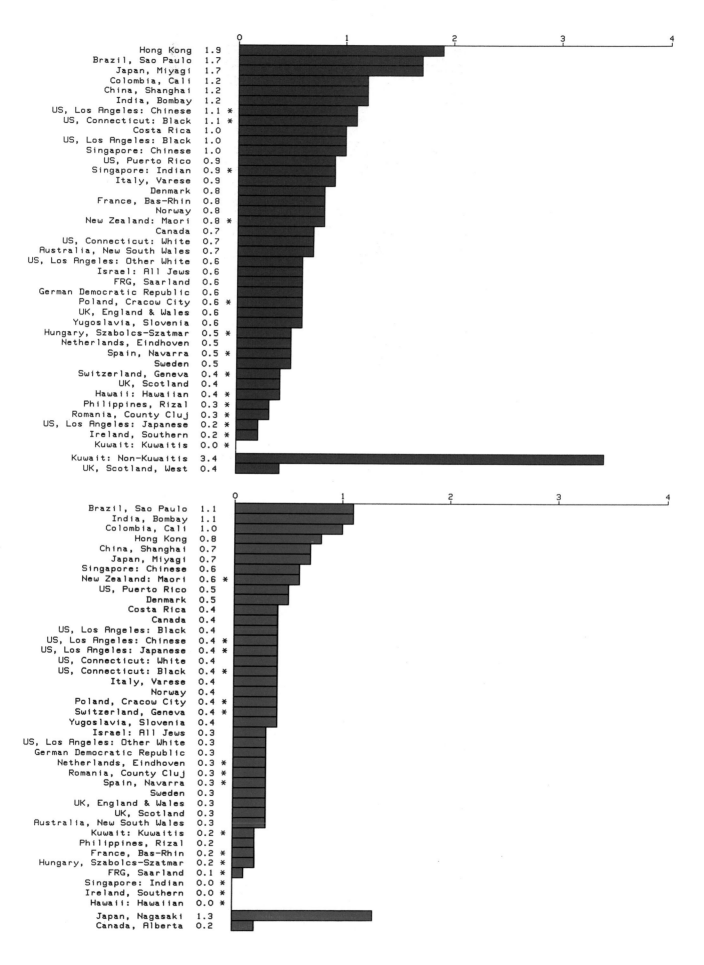

* Rates based on less than 10 cases

161 LARYNX

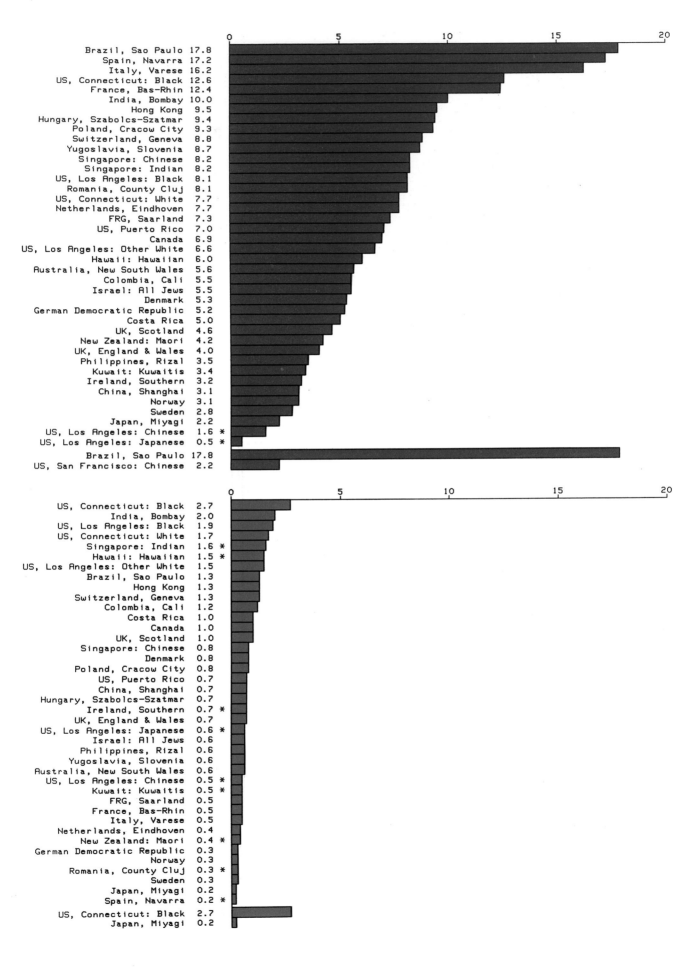

Brazil, Sao Paulo	17.8
Spain, Navarra	17.2
Italy, Varese	16.2
US, Connecticut: Black	12.6
France, Bas-Rhin	12.4
India, Bombay	10.0
Hong Kong	9.5
Hungary, Szabolcs-Szatmar	9.4
Poland, Cracow City	9.3
Switzerland, Geneva	8.8
Yugoslavia, Slovenia	8.7
Singapore: Chinese	8.2
Singapore: Indian	8.2
US, Los Angeles: Black	8.1
Romania, County Cluj	8.1
US, Connecticut: White	7.7
Netherlands, Eindhoven	7.7
FRG, Saarland	7.3
US, Puerto Rico	7.0
Canada	6.9
US, Los Angeles: Other White	6.6
Hawaii: Hawaiian	6.0
Australia, New South Wales	5.6
Colombia, Cali	5.5
Israel: All Jews	5.5
Denmark	5.3
German Democratic Republic	5.2
Costa Rica	5.0
UK, Scotland	4.6
New Zealand: Maori	4.2
UK, England & Wales	4.0
Philippines, Rizal	3.5
Kuwait: Kuwaitis	3.4
Ireland, Southern	3.2
China, Shanghai	3.1
Norway	3.1
Sweden	2.8
Japan, Miyagi	2.2
US, Los Angeles: Chinese	1.6 *
US, Los Angeles: Japanese	0.5 *
Brazil, Sao Paulo	17.8
US, San Francisco: Chinese	2.2

US, Connecticut: Black	2.7
India, Bombay	2.0
US, Los Angeles: Black	1.9
US, Connecticut: White	1.7
Singapore: Indian	1.6 *
Hawaii: Hawaiian	1.5 *
US, Los Angeles: Other White	1.5
Brazil, Sao Paulo	1.3
Hong Kong	1.3
Switzerland, Geneva	1.3
Colombia, Cali	1.2
Costa Rica	1.0
Canada	1.0
UK, Scotland	1.0
Singapore: Chinese	0.8
Denmark	0.8
Poland, Cracow City	0.8
US, Puerto Rico	0.7
China, Shanghai	0.7
Hungary, Szabolcs-Szatmar	0.7
Ireland, Southern	0.7 *
UK, England & Wales	0.7
US, Los Angeles: Japanese	0.6 *
Israel: All Jews	0.6
Philippines, Rizal	0.6
Yugoslavia, Slovenia	0.6
Australia, New South Wales	0.6
US, Los Angeles: Chinese	0.5 *
Kuwait: Kuwaitis	0.5 *
FRG, Saarland	0.5
France, Bas-Rhin	0.5
Italy, Varese	0.5
Netherlands, Eindhoven	0.4
New Zealand: Maori	0.4 *
German Democratic Republic	0.3
Norway	0.3
Romania, County Cluj	0.3 *
Sweden	0.3
Japan, Miyagi	0.2
Spain, Navarra	0.2 *
US, Connecticut: Black	2.7
Japan, Miyagi	0.2

* Rates based on less than 10 cases

162 BRONCHUS, LUNG

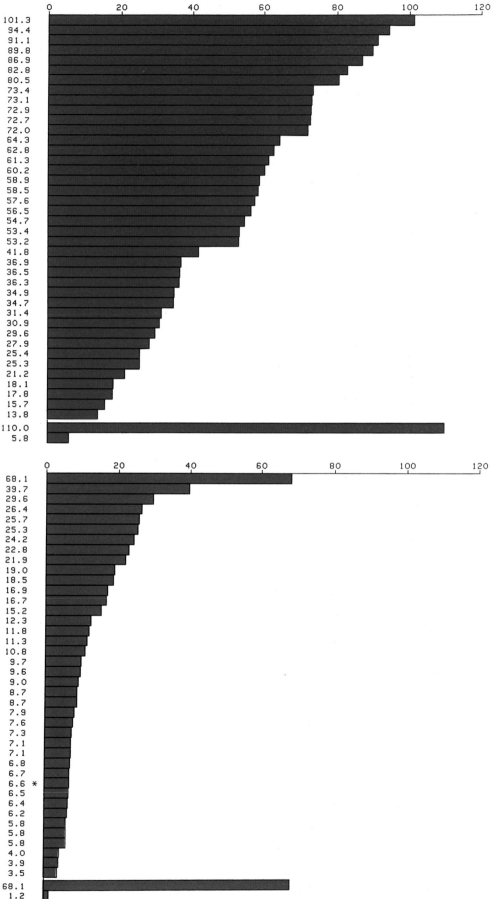

New Zealand: Maori	101.3
Netherlands, Eindhoven	94.4
UK, Scotland	91.1
US, Connecticut: Black	89.8
US, Los Angeles: Black	86.9
Hawaii: Hawaiian	82.8
Italy, Varese	80.5
Singapore: Chinese	73.4
Poland, Cracow City	73.1
Switzerland, Geneva	72.9
FRG, Saarland	72.7
UK, England & Wales	72.0
US, Connecticut: White	64.3
US, Los Angeles: Other White	62.8
Canada	61.3
France, Bas-Rhin	60.2
German Democratic Republic	58.9
Hong Kong	58.5
Yugoslavia, Slovenia	57.6
Denmark	56.5
China, Shanghai	54.7
Australia, New South Wales	53.4
Hungary, Szabolcs-Szatmar	53.2
US, Los Angeles: Chinese	41.8
Philippines, Rizal	36.9
Brazil, Sao Paulo	36.5
Ireland, Southern	36.3
Spain, Navarra	34.9
Romania, County Cluj	34.7
US, Los Angeles: Japanese	31.4
Norway	30.9
Japan, Miyagi	29.6
Israel: All Jews	27.9
Colombia, Cali	25.4
Sweden	25.3
Singapore: Indian	21.2
US, Puerto Rico	18.1
Costa Rica	17.8
India, Bombay	15.7
Kuwait: Kuwaitis	13.8
US, New Orleans: Black	110.0
India, Madras	5.8

New Zealand: Maori	68.1
Hawaii: Hawaiian	39.7
US, Los Angeles: Other White	29.6
UK, Scotland	26.4
US, Los Angeles: Black	25.7
US, Connecticut: White	25.3
Hong Kong	24.2
Singapore: Chinese	22.8
US, Connecticut: Black	21.9
UK, England & Wales	19.0
China, Shanghai	18.5
Canada	16.9
Denmark	16.7
US, Los Angeles: Chinese	15.2
Poland, Cracow City	12.3
Ireland, Southern	11.8
Australia, New South Wales	11.3
Switzerland, Geneva	10.8
Colombia, Cali	9.7
US, Los Angeles: Japanese	9.6
Israel: All Jews	9.0
Japan, Miyagi	8.7
Philippines, Rizal	8.7
Brazil, Sao Paulo	7.9
Sweden	7.6
Norway	7.3
FRG, Saarland	7.1
Hungary, Szabolcs-Szatmar	7.1
Costa Rica	6.8
Yugoslavia, Slovenia	6.7
Singapore: Indian	6.6 *
US, Puerto Rico	6.5
Kuwait: Kuwaitis	6.4
Italy, Varese	6.2
German Democratic Republic	5.8
Netherlands, Eindhoven	5.8
Romania, County Cluj	5.8
Spain, Navarra	4.0
France, Bas-Rhin	3.9
India, Bombay	3.5
New Zealand: Maori	68.1
India, Madras	1.2

* Rates based on less than 10 cases

25

163 PLEURA

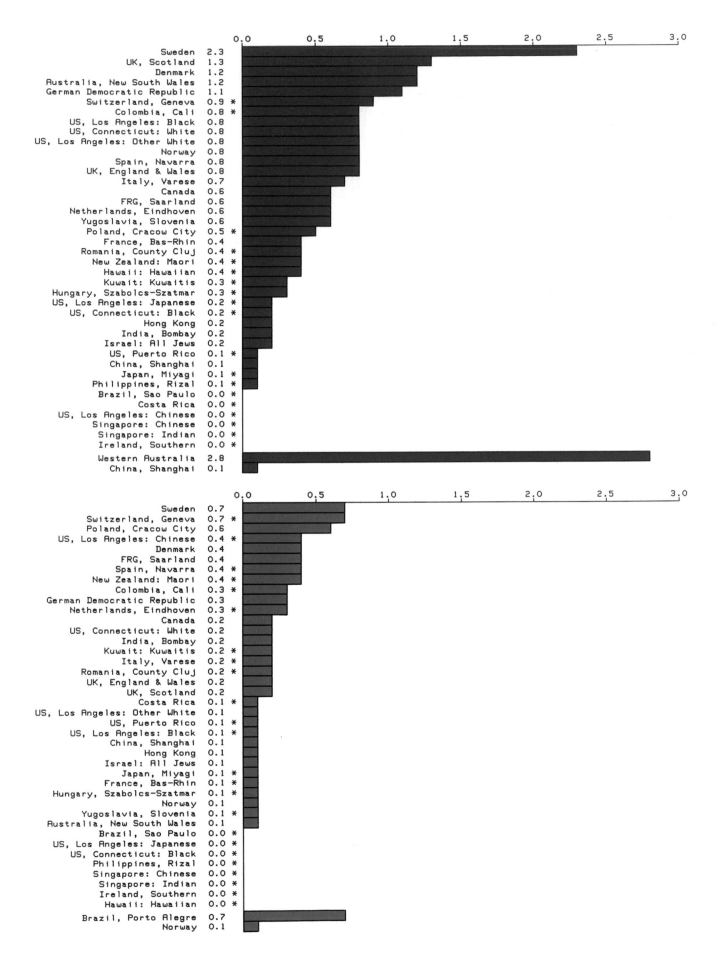

* Rates based on less than 10 cases

170 BONE

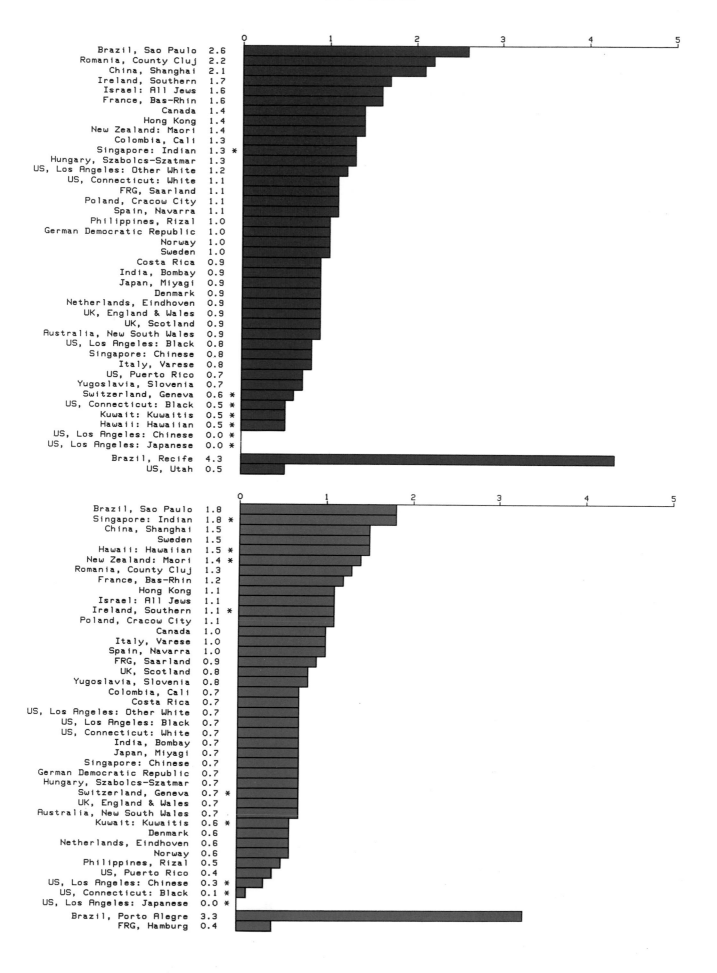

171 CONNECTIVE TISSUE

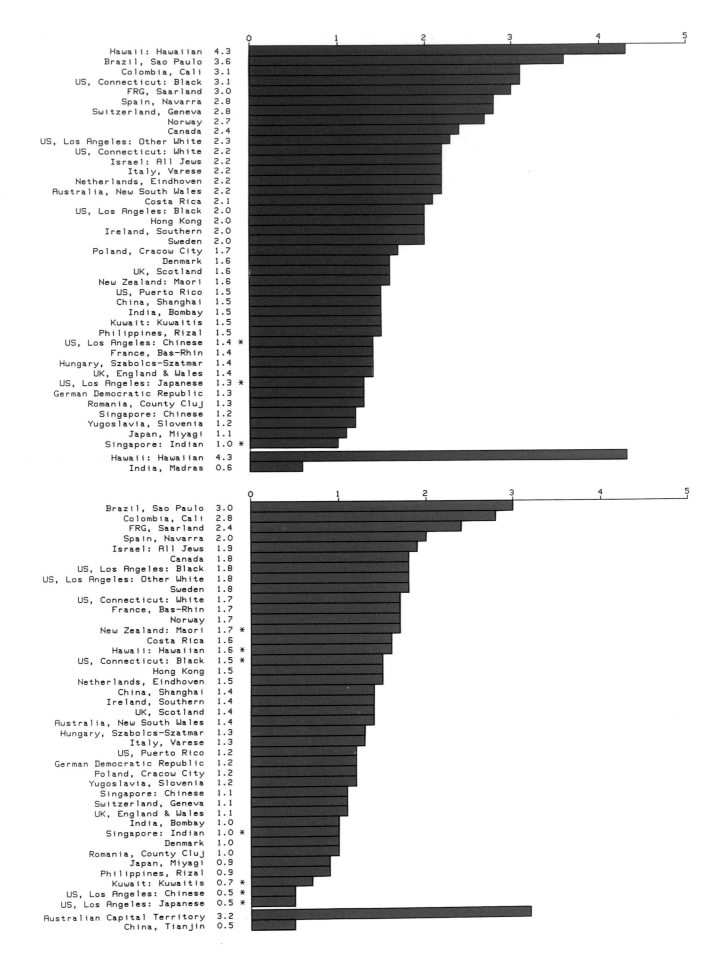

Hawaii: Hawaiian 4.3
Brazil, Sao Paulo 3.6
Colombia, Cali 3.1
US, Connecticut: Black 3.1
FRG, Saarland 3.0
Spain, Navarra 2.8
Switzerland, Geneva 2.8
Norway 2.7
Canada 2.4
US, Los Angeles: Other White 2.3
US, Connecticut: White 2.2
Israel: All Jews 2.2
Italy, Varese 2.2
Netherlands, Eindhoven 2.2
Australia, New South Wales 2.2
Costa Rica 2.1
US, Los Angeles: Black 2.0
Hong Kong 2.0
Ireland, Southern 2.0
Sweden 2.0
Poland, Cracow City 1.7
Denmark 1.6
UK, Scotland 1.6
New Zealand: Maori 1.6
US, Puerto Rico 1.5
China, Shanghai 1.5
India, Bombay 1.5
Kuwait: Kuwaitis 1.5
Philippines, Rizal 1.5
US, Los Angeles: Chinese 1.4 *
France, Bas-Rhin 1.4
Hungary, Szabolcs-Szatmar 1.4
UK, England & Wales 1.4
US, Los Angeles: Japanese 1.3 *
German Democratic Republic 1.3
Romania, County Cluj 1.3
Singapore: Chinese 1.2
Yugoslavia, Slovenia 1.2
Japan, Miyagi 1.1
Singapore: Indian 1.0 *

Hawaii: Hawaiian 4.3
India, Madras 0.6

Brazil, Sao Paulo 3.0
Colombia, Cali 2.8
FRG, Saarland 2.4
Spain, Navarra 2.0
Israel: All Jews 1.9
Canada 1.8
US, Los Angeles: Black 1.8
US, Los Angeles: Other White 1.8
Sweden 1.8
US, Connecticut: White 1.7
France, Bas-Rhin 1.7
Norway 1.7
New Zealand: Maori 1.7 *
Costa Rica 1.6
Hawaii: Hawaiian 1.6 *
US, Connecticut: Black 1.5 *
Hong Kong 1.5
Netherlands, Eindhoven 1.5
China, Shanghai 1.4
Ireland, Southern 1.4
UK, Scotland 1.4
Australia, New South Wales 1.4
Hungary, Szabolcs-Szatmar 1.3
Italy, Varese 1.3
US, Puerto Rico 1.2
German Democratic Republic 1.2
Poland, Cracow City 1.2
Yugoslavia, Slovenia 1.2
Singapore: Chinese 1.1
Switzerland, Geneva 1.1
UK, England & Wales 1.1
India, Bombay 1.0
Singapore: Indian 1.0 *
Denmark 1.0
Romania, County Cluj 1.0
Japan, Miyagi 0.9
Philippines, Rizal 0.9
Kuwait: Kuwaitis 0.7 *
US, Los Angeles: Chinese 0.5 *
US, Los Angeles: Japanese 0.5 *

Australian Capital Territory 3.2
China, Tianjin 0.5

* Rates based on less than 10 cases

28

172 MELANOMA OF SKIN

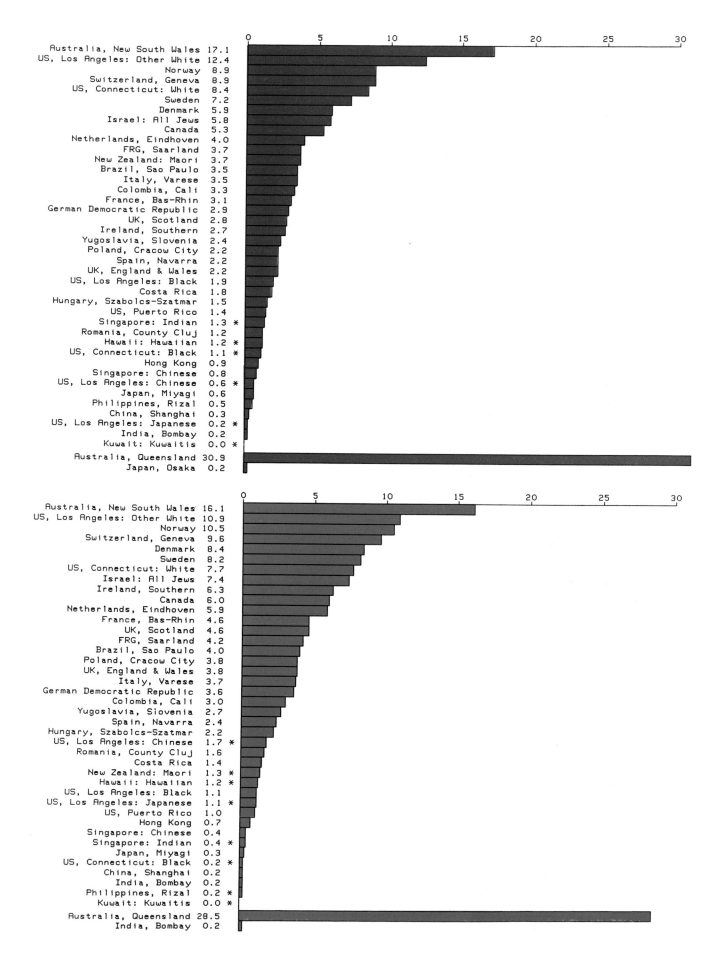

Australia, New South Wales	17.1
US, Los Angeles: Other White	12.4
Norway	8.9
Switzerland, Geneva	8.9
US, Connecticut: White	8.4
Sweden	7.2
Denmark	5.9
Israel: All Jews	5.8
Canada	5.3
Netherlands, Eindhoven	4.0
FRG, Saarland	3.7
New Zealand: Maori	3.7
Brazil, Sao Paulo	3.5
Italy, Varese	3.5
Colombia, Cali	3.3
France, Bas-Rhin	3.1
German Democratic Republic	2.9
UK, Scotland	2.8
Ireland, Southern	2.7
Yugoslavia, Slovenia	2.4
Poland, Cracow City	2.2
Spain, Navarra	2.2
UK, England & Wales	2.2
US, Los Angeles: Black	1.9
Costa Rica	1.8
Hungary, Szabolcs-Szatmar	1.5
US, Puerto Rico	1.4
Singapore: Indian	1.3 *
Romania, County Cluj	1.2
Hawaii: Hawaiian	1.2 *
US, Connecticut: Black	1.1 *
Hong Kong	0.9
Singapore: Chinese	0.8
US, Los Angeles: Chinese	0.6 *
Japan, Miyagi	0.6
Philippines, Rizal	0.5
China, Shanghai	0.3
US, Los Angeles: Japanese	0.2 *
India, Bombay	0.2
Kuwait: Kuwaitis	0.0 *
Australia, Queensland	30.9
Japan, Osaka	0.2

Australia, New South Wales	16.1
US, Los Angeles: Other White	10.9
Norway	10.5
Switzerland, Geneva	9.6
Denmark	8.4
Sweden	8.2
US, Connecticut: White	7.7
Israel: All Jews	7.4
Ireland, Southern	6.3
Canada	6.0
Netherlands, Eindhoven	5.9
France, Bas-Rhin	4.6
UK, Scotland	4.6
FRG, Saarland	4.2
Brazil, Sao Paulo	4.0
Poland, Cracow City	3.8
UK, England & Wales	3.8
Italy, Varese	3.7
German Democratic Republic	3.6
Colombia, Cali	3.0
Yugoslavia, Slovenia	2.7
Spain, Navarra	2.4
Hungary, Szabolcs-Szatmar	2.2
US, Los Angeles: Chinese	1.7 *
Romania, County Cluj	1.6
Costa Rica	1.4
New Zealand: Maori	1.3 *
Hawaii: Hawaiian	1.2 *
US, Los Angeles: Black	1.1
US, Los Angeles: Japanese	1.1 *
US, Puerto Rico	1.0
Hong Kong	0.7
Singapore: Chinese	0.4
Singapore: Indian	0.4 *
Japan, Miyagi	0.3
US, Connecticut: Black	0.2 *
China, Shanghai	0.2
India, Bombay	0.2
Philippines, Rizal	0.2 *
Kuwait: Kuwaitis	0.0 *
Australia, Queensland	28.5
India, Bombay	0.2

* Rates based on less than 10 cases

29

174-5 BREAST

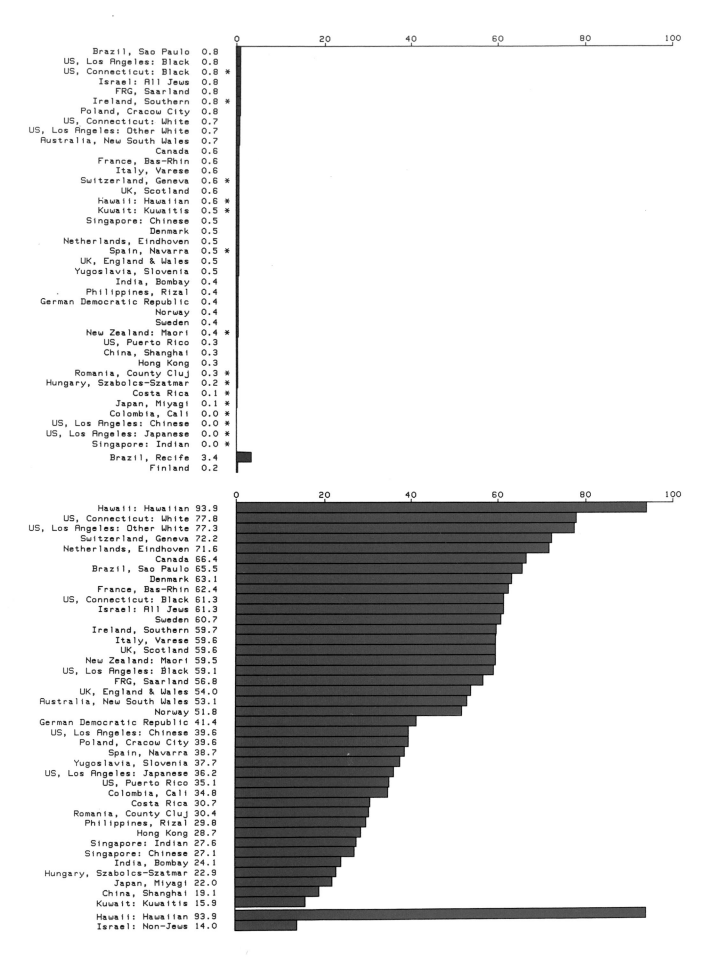

Brazil, Sao Paulo	0.8
US, Los Angeles: Black	0.8
US, Connecticut: Black	0.8 *
Israel: All Jews	0.8
FRG, Saarland	0.8
Ireland, Southern	0.8 *
Poland, Cracow City	0.8
US, Connecticut: White	0.7
US, Los Angeles: Other White	0.7
Australia, New South Wales	0.7
Canada	0.6
France, Bas-Rhin	0.6
Italy, Varese	0.6
Switzerland, Geneva	0.6 *
UK, Scotland	0.6
Hawaii: Hawaiian	0.6 *
Kuwait: Kuwaitis	0.5 *
Singapore: Chinese	0.5
Denmark	0.5
Netherlands, Eindhoven	0.5
Spain, Navarra	0.5 *
UK, England & Wales	0.5
Yugoslavia, Slovenia	0.5
India, Bombay	0.4
Philippines, Rizal	0.4
German Democratic Republic	0.4
Norway	0.4
Sweden	0.4
New Zealand: Maori	0.4 *
US, Puerto Rico	0.3
China, Shanghai	0.3
Hong Kong	0.3
Romania, County Cluj	0.3 *
Hungary, Szabolcs-Szatmar	0.2 *
Costa Rica	0.1 *
Japan, Miyagi	0.1 *
Colombia, Cali	0.0 *
US, Los Angeles: Chinese	0.0 *
US, Los Angeles: Japanese	0.0 *
Singapore: Indian	0.0 *
Brazil, Recife	3.4
Finland	0.2

Hawaii: Hawaiian	93.9
US, Connecticut: White	77.8
US, Los Angeles: Other White	77.3
Switzerland, Geneva	72.2
Netherlands, Eindhoven	71.6
Canada	66.4
Brazil, Sao Paulo	65.5
Denmark	63.1
France, Bas-Rhin	62.4
US, Connecticut: Black	61.3
Israel: All Jews	61.3
Sweden	60.7
Ireland, Southern	59.7
Italy, Varese	59.6
UK, Scotland	59.6
New Zealand: Maori	59.5
US, Los Angeles: Black	59.1
FRG, Saarland	56.8
UK, England & Wales	54.0
Australia, New South Wales	53.1
Norway	51.8
German Democratic Republic	41.4
US, Los Angeles: Chinese	39.6
Poland, Cracow City	39.6
Spain, Navarra	38.7
Yugoslavia, Slovenia	37.7
US, Los Angeles: Japanese	36.2
US, Puerto Rico	35.1
Colombia, Cali	34.8
Costa Rica	30.7
Romania, County Cluj	30.4
Philippines, Rizal	29.8
Hong Kong	28.7
Singapore: Indian	27.6
Singapore: Chinese	27.1
India, Bombay	24.1
Hungary, Szabolcs-Szatmar	22.9
Japan, Miyagi	22.0
China, Shanghai	19.1
Kuwait: Kuwaitis	15.9
Hawaii: Hawaiian	93.9
Israel: Non-Jews	14.0

* Rates based on less than 10 cases

180 CERVIX UTERI

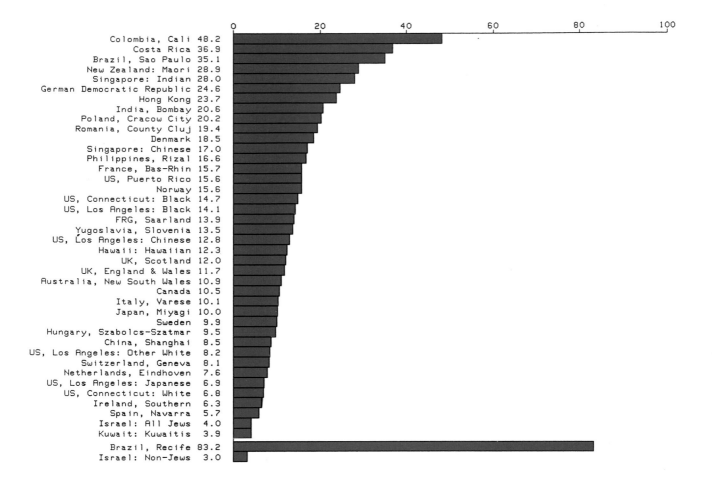

Colombia, Cali	48.2
Costa Rica	36.9
Brazil, Sao Paulo	35.1
New Zealand: Maori	28.9
Singapore: Indian	28.0
German Democratic Republic	24.6
Hong Kong	23.7
India, Bombay	20.6
Poland, Cracow City	20.2
Romania, County Cluj	19.4
Denmark	18.5
Singapore: Chinese	17.0
Philippines, Rizal	16.6
France, Bas-Rhin	15.7
US, Puerto Rico	15.6
Norway	15.6
US, Connecticut: Black	14.7
US, Los Angeles: Black	14.1
FRG, Saarland	13.9
Yugoslavia, Slovenia	13.5
US, Los Angeles: Chinese	12.8
Hawaii: Hawaiian	12.3
UK, Scotland	12.0
UK, England & Wales	11.7
Australia, New South Wales	10.9
Canada	10.5
Italy, Varese	10.1
Japan, Miyagi	10.0
Sweden	9.9
Hungary, Szabolcs-Szatmar	9.5
China, Shanghai	8.5
US, Los Angeles: Other White	8.2
Switzerland, Geneva	8.1
Netherlands, Eindhoven	7.6
US, Los Angeles: Japanese	6.9
US, Connecticut: White	6.8
Ireland, Southern	6.3
Spain, Navarra	5.7
Israel: All Jews	4.0
Kuwait: Kuwaitis	3.9
Brazil, Recife	83.2
Israel: Non-Jews	3.0

181 PLACENTA

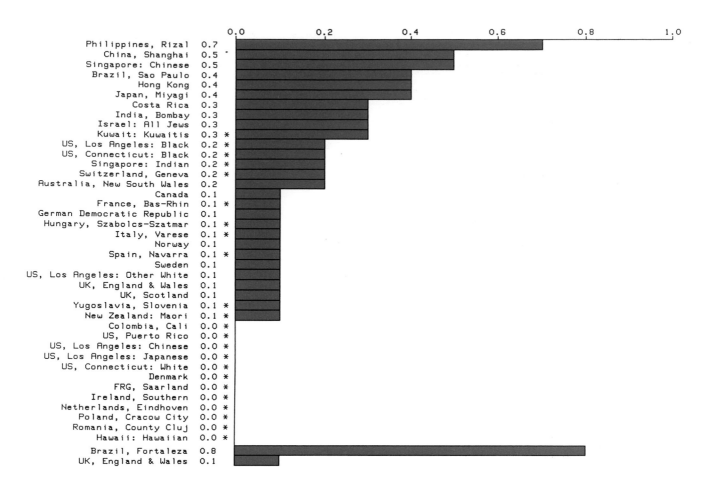

Philippines, Rizal 0.7
China, Shanghai 0.5
Singapore: Chinese 0.5
Brazil, Sao Paulo 0.4
Hong Kong 0.4
Japan, Miyagi 0.4
Costa Rica 0.3
India, Bombay 0.3
Israel: All Jews 0.3
Kuwait: Kuwaitis 0.3 *
US, Los Angeles: Black 0.2 *
US, Connecticut: Black 0.2 *
Singapore: Indian 0.2 *
Switzerland, Geneva 0.2 *
Australia, New South Wales 0.2
Canada 0.1
France, Bas-Rhin 0.1 *
German Democratic Republic 0.1
Hungary, Szabolcs-Szatmar 0.1 *
Italy, Varese 0.1 *
Norway 0.1
Spain, Navarra 0.1 *
Sweden 0.1
US, Los Angeles: Other White 0.1
UK, England & Wales 0.1
UK, Scotland 0.1
Yugoslavia, Slovenia 0.1 *
New Zealand: Maori 0.1 *
Colombia, Cali 0.0 *
US, Puerto Rico 0.0 *
US, Los Angeles: Chinese 0.0 *
US, Los Angeles: Japanese 0.0 *
US, Connecticut: White 0.0 *
Denmark 0.0 *
FRG, Saarland 0.0 *
Ireland, Southern 0.0 *
Netherlands, Eindhoven 0.0 *
Poland, Cracow City 0.0 *
Romania, County Cluj 0.0 *
Hawaii: Hawaiian 0.0 *

Brazil, Fortaleza 0.8
UK, England & Wales 0.1

* Rates based on less than 10 cases

182 CORPUS UTERI

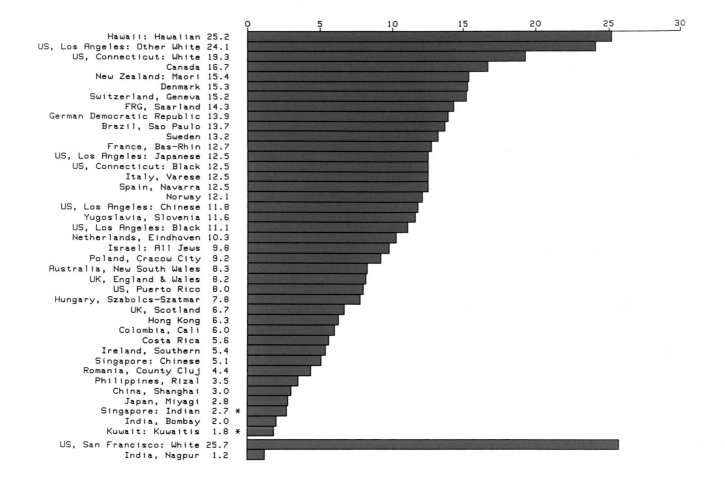

Hawaii: Hawaiian	25.2
US, Los Angeles: Other White	24.1
US, Connecticut: White	19.3
Canada	16.7
New Zealand: Maori	15.4
Denmark	15.3
Switzerland, Geneva	15.2
FRG, Saarland	14.3
German Democratic Republic	13.9
Brazil, Sao Paulo	13.7
Sweden	13.2
France, Bas-Rhin	12.7
US, Los Angeles: Japanese	12.5
US, Connecticut: Black	12.5
Italy, Varese	12.5
Spain, Navarra	12.5
Norway	12.1
US, Los Angeles: Chinese	11.8
Yugoslavia, Slovenia	11.6
US, Los Angeles: Black	11.1
Netherlands, Eindhoven	10.3
Israel: All Jews	9.8
Poland, Cracow City	9.2
Australia, New South Wales	8.3
UK, England & Wales	8.2
US, Puerto Rico	8.0
Hungary, Szabolcs-Szatmar	7.8
UK, Scotland	6.7
Hong Kong	6.3
Colombia, Cali	6.0
Costa Rica	5.6
Ireland, Southern	5.4
Singapore: Chinese	5.1
Romania, County Cluj	4.4
Philippines, Rizal	3.5
China, Shanghai	3.0
Japan, Miyagi	2.8
Singapore: Indian	2.7 *
India, Bombay	2.0
Kuwait: Kuwaitis	1.8 *
US, San Francisco: White	25.7
India, Nagpur	1.2

* Rates based on less than 10 cases

33

183 OVARY ETC.

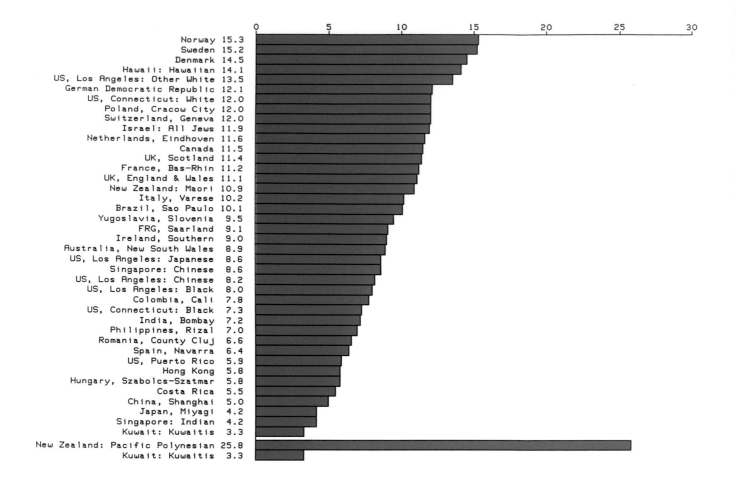

Country	Value
Norway	15.3
Sweden	15.2
Denmark	14.5
Hawaii: Hawaiian	14.1
US, Los Angeles: Other White	13.5
German Democratic Republic	12.1
US, Connecticut: White	12.0
Poland, Cracow City	12.0
Switzerland, Geneva	12.0
Israel: All Jews	11.9
Netherlands, Eindhoven	11.6
Canada	11.5
UK, Scotland	11.4
France, Bas-Rhin	11.2
UK, England & Wales	11.1
New Zealand: Maori	10.9
Italy, Varese	10.2
Brazil, Sao Paulo	10.1
Yugoslavia, Slovenia	9.5
FRG, Saarland	9.1
Ireland, Southern	9.0
Australia, New South Wales	8.9
US, Los Angeles: Japanese	8.6
Singapore: Chinese	8.6
US, Los Angeles: Chinese	8.2
US, Los Angeles: Black	8.0
Colombia, Cali	7.8
US, Connecticut: Black	7.3
India, Bombay	7.2
Philippines, Rizal	7.0
Romania, County Cluj	6.6
Spain, Navarra	6.4
US, Puerto Rico	5.9
Hong Kong	5.8
Hungary, Szabolcs-Szatmar	5.8
Costa Rica	5.5
China, Shanghai	5.0
Japan, Miyagi	4.2
Singapore: Indian	4.2
Kuwait: Kuwaitis	3.3
New Zealand: Pacific Polynesian	25.8
Kuwait: Kuwaitis	3.3

34

184 OTHER FEMALE GENITAL

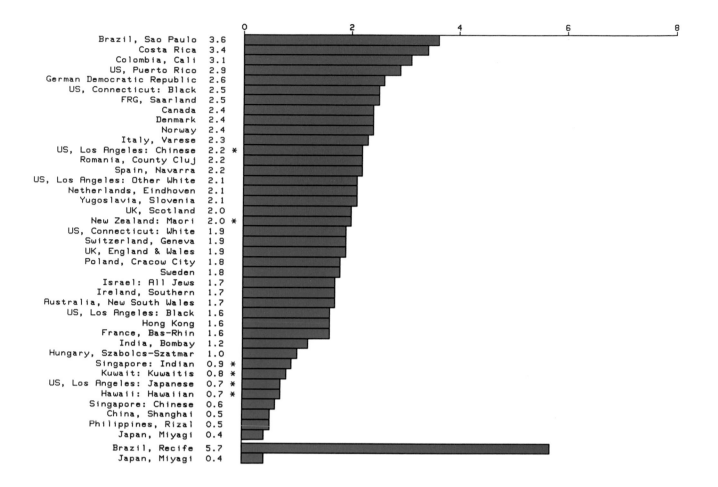

Brazil, Sao Paulo	3.6
Costa Rica	3.4
Colombia, Cali	3.1
US, Puerto Rico	2.9
German Democratic Republic	2.6
US, Connecticut: Black	2.5
FRG, Saarland	2.5
Canada	2.4
Denmark	2.4
Norway	2.4
Italy, Varese	2.3
US, Los Angeles: Chinese	2.2 *
Romania, County Cluj	2.2
Spain, Navarra	2.2
US, Los Angeles: Other White	2.1
Netherlands, Eindhoven	2.1
Yugoslavia, Slovenia	2.1
UK, Scotland	2.0
New Zealand: Maori	2.0 *
US, Connecticut: White	1.9
Switzerland, Geneva	1.9
UK, England & Wales	1.9
Poland, Cracow City	1.8
Sweden	1.8
Israel: All Jews	1.7
Ireland, Southern	1.7
Australia, New South Wales	1.7
US, Los Angeles: Black	1.6
Hong Kong	1.6
France, Bas-Rhin	1.6
India, Bombay	1.2
Hungary, Szabolcs-Szatmar	1.0
Singapore: Indian	0.9 *
Kuwait: Kuwaitis	0.8 *
US, Los Angeles: Japanese	0.7 *
Hawaii: Hawaiian	0.7 *
Singapore: Chinese	0.6
China, Shanghai	0.5
Philippines, Rizal	0.5
Japan, Miyagi	0.4
Brazil, Recife	5.7
Japan, Miyagi	0.4

* Rates based on less than 10 cases

185 PROSTATE

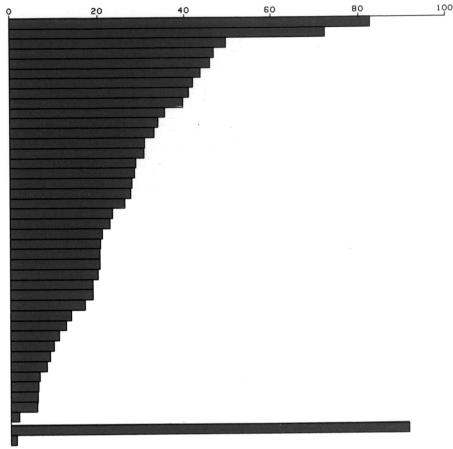

US, Los Angeles: Black	82.6
US, Connecticut: Black	72.3
US, Los Angeles: Other White	49.6
US, Connecticut: White	46.8
Sweden	45.9
Canada	43.7
Norway	42.0
Hawaii: Hawaiian	40.9
Switzerland, Geneva	39.6
New Zealand: Maori	35.4
Australia, New South Wales	33.8
Brazil, Sao Paulo	33.0
US, Puerto Rico	30.7
Colombia, Cali	30.6
FRG, Saarland	28.7
Netherlands, Eindhoven	28.3
Denmark	27.7
France, Bas-Rhin	27.4
Costa Rica	26.1
UK, Scotland	23.3
US, Los Angeles: Japanese	22.8
UK, England & Wales	20.9
Spain, Navarra	20.5
Ireland, Southern	20.3
Italy, Varese	20.3
German Democratic Republic	19.9
Israel: All Jews	18.8
Yugoslavia, Slovenia	18.7
US, Los Angeles: Chinese	16.9
Poland, Cracow City	13.8
Hungary, Szabolcs-Szatmar	12.6
Philippines, Rizal	11.1
Romania, County Cluj	9.8
Singapore: Indian	8.9
India, Bombay	8.2
Singapore: Chinese	6.6
Japan, Miyagi	6.3
Hong Kong	6.2
Kuwait: Kuwaitis	6.0
China, Shanghai	1.8
US, Atlanta: Black	91.2
China, Tianjin	1.3

186 TESTIS

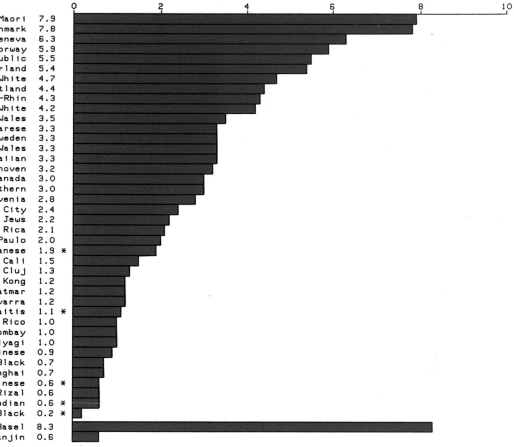

		0	2	4	6	8	10
New Zealand: Maori	7.9						
Denmark	7.8						
Switzerland, Geneva	6.3						
Norway	5.9						
German Democratic Republic	5.5						
FRG, Saarland	5.4						
US, Los Angeles: Other White	4.7						
UK, Scotland	4.4						
France, Bas-Rhin	4.3						
US, Connecticut: White	4.2						
Australia, New South Wales	3.5						
Italy, Varese	3.3						
Sweden	3.3						
UK, England & Wales	3.3						
Hawaii: Hawaiian	3.3						
Netherlands, Eindhoven	3.2						
Canada	3.0						
Ireland, Southern	3.0						
Yugoslavia, Slovenia	2.8						
Poland, Cracow City	2.4						
Israel: All Jews	2.2						
Costa Rica	2.1						
Brazil, Sao Paulo	2.0						
US, Los Angeles: Japanese	1.9 *						
Colombia, Cali	1.5						
Romania, County Cluj	1.3						
Hong Kong	1.2						
Hungary, Szabolcs-Szatmar	1.2						
Spain, Navarra	1.2						
Kuwait: Kuwaitis	1.1 *						
US, Puerto Rico	1.0						
India, Bombay	1.0						
Japan, Miyagi	1.0						
Singapore: Chinese	0.9						
US, Los Angeles: Black	0.7						
China, Shanghai	0.7						
US, Los Angeles: Chinese	0.6 *						
Philippines, Rizal	0.6						
Singapore: Indian	0.6 *						
US, Connecticut: Black	0.2 *						
Switzerland, Basel	8.3						
China, Tianjin	0.6						

* Rates based on less than 10 cases

37

187.1-.4 PENIS

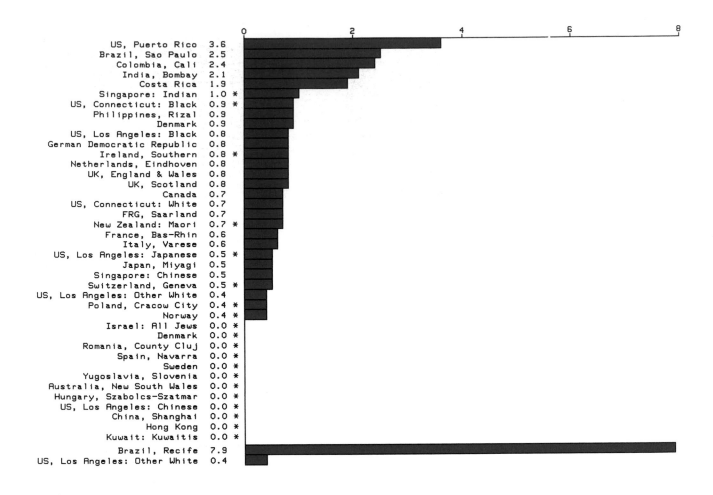

US, Puerto Rico	3.6
Brazil, Sao Paulo	2.5
Colombia, Cali	2.4
India, Bombay	2.1
Costa Rica	1.9
Singapore: Indian	1.0 *
US, Connecticut: Black	0.9 *
Philippines, Rizal	0.9
Denmark	0.9
US, Los Angeles: Black	0.8
German Democratic Republic	0.8
Ireland, Southern	0.8 *
Netherlands, Eindhoven	0.8
UK, England & Wales	0.8
UK, Scotland	0.8
Canada	0.7
US, Connecticut: White	0.7
FRG, Saarland	0.7
New Zealand: Maori	0.7 *
France, Bas-Rhin	0.6
Italy, Varese	0.6
US, Los Angeles: Japanese	0.5 *
Japan, Miyagi	0.5
Singapore: Chinese	0.5
Switzerland, Geneva	0.5 *
US, Los Angeles: Other White	0.4
Poland, Cracow City	0.4 *
Norway	0.4 *
Israel: All Jews	0.0 *
Denmark	0.0 *
Romania, County Cluj	0.0 *
Spain, Navarra	0.0 *
Sweden	0.0 *
Yugoslavia, Slovenia	0.0 *
Australia, New South Wales	0.0 *
Hungary, Szabolcs-Szatmar	0.0 *
US, Los Angeles: Chinese	0.0 *
China, Shanghai	0.0 *
Hong Kong	0.0 *
Kuwait: Kuwaitis	0.0 *
Brazil, Recife	7.9
US, Los Angeles: Other White	0.4

* Rates based on less than 10 cases

188 BLADDER

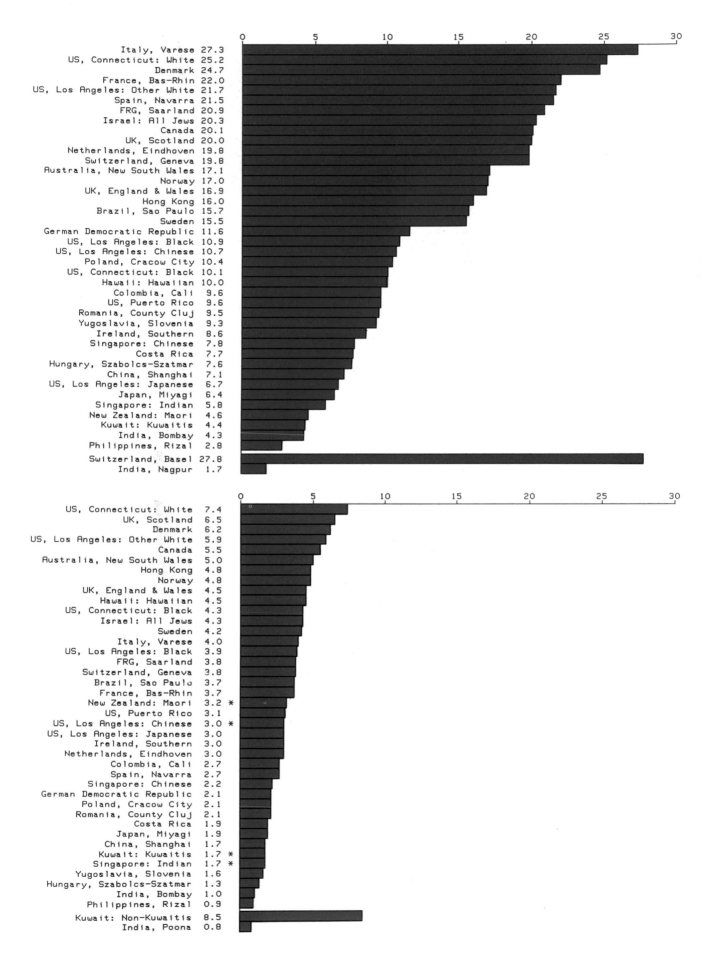

Italy, Varese	27.3
US, Connecticut: White	25.2
Denmark	24.7
France, Bas-Rhin	22.0
US, Los Angeles: Other White	21.7
Spain, Navarra	21.5
FRG, Saarland	20.9
Israel: All Jews	20.3
Canada	20.1
UK, Scotland	20.0
Netherlands, Eindhoven	19.8
Switzerland, Geneva	19.8
Australia, New South Wales	17.1
Norway	17.0
UK, England & Wales	16.9
Hong Kong	16.0
Brazil, Sao Paulo	15.7
Sweden	15.5
German Democratic Republic	11.6
US, Los Angeles: Black	10.9
US, Los Angeles: Chinese	10.7
Poland, Cracow City	10.4
US, Connecticut: Black	10.1
Hawaii: Hawaiian	10.0
Colombia, Cali	9.6
US, Puerto Rico	9.6
Romania, County Cluj	9.5
Yugoslavia, Slovenia	9.3
Ireland, Southern	8.6
Singapore: Chinese	7.8
Costa Rica	7.7
Hungary, Szabolcs-Szatmar	7.6
China, Shanghai	7.1
US, Los Angeles: Japanese	6.7
Japan, Miyagi	6.4
Singapore: Indian	5.8
New Zealand: Maori	4.6
Kuwait: Kuwaitis	4.4
India, Bombay	4.3
Philippines, Rizal	2.8
Switzerland, Basel	27.8
India, Nagpur	1.7

US, Connecticut: White	7.4
UK, Scotland	6.5
Denmark	6.2
US, Los Angeles: Other White	5.9
Canada	5.5
Australia, New South Wales	5.0
Hong Kong	4.8
Norway	4.8
UK, England & Wales	4.5
Hawaii: Hawaiian	4.5
US, Connecticut: Black	4.3
Israel: All Jews	4.3
Sweden	4.2
Italy, Varese	4.0
US, Los Angeles: Black	3.9
FRG, Saarland	3.8
Switzerland, Geneva	3.8
Brazil, Sao Paulo	3.7
France, Bas-Rhin	3.7
New Zealand: Maori	3.2 *
US, Puerto Rico	3.1
US, Los Angeles: Chinese	3.0 *
US, Los Angeles: Japanese	3.0
Ireland, Southern	3.0
Netherlands, Eindhoven	3.0
Colombia, Cali	2.7
Spain, Navarra	2.7
Singapore: Chinese	2.2
German Democratic Republic	2.1
Poland, Cracow City	2.1
Romania, County Cluj	2.1
Costa Rica	1.9
Japan, Miyagi	1.9
China, Shanghai	1.7
Kuwait: Kuwaitis	1.7 *
Singapore: Indian	1.7 *
Yugoslavia, Slovenia	1.6
Hungary, Szabolcs-Szatmar	1.3
India, Bombay	1.0
Philippines, Rizal	0.9
Kuwait: Non-Kuwaitis	8.5
India, Poona	0.8

* Rates based on less than 10 cases

39

189 OTHER URINARY

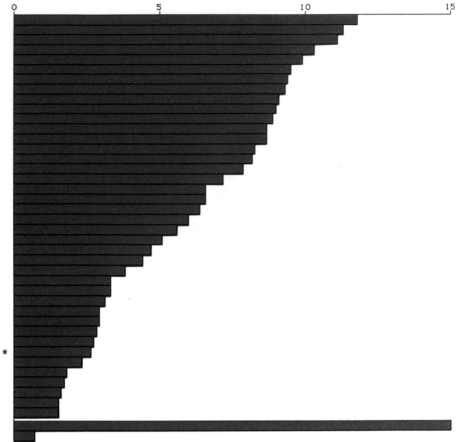

US, Connecticut: Black	11.8
Sweden	11.3
France, Bas-Rhin	11.1
FRG, Saarland	10.3
US, Connecticut: White	9.9
Switzerland, Geneva	9.5
Denmark	9.4
Italy, Varese	9.3
Netherlands, Eindhoven	9.1
US, Los Angeles: Other White	9.0
Norway	8.9
US, Los Angeles: Black	8.7
German Democratic Republic	8.7
US, Los Angeles: Chinese	8.3
Hawaii: Hawaiian	8.2
Canada	7.9
Australia, New South Wales	7.2
Israel: All Jews	6.6
UK, Scotland	6.6
Poland, Cracow City	6.4
New Zealand: Maori	6.0
Spain, Navarra	5.6
UK, England & Wales	5.1
Yugoslavia, Slovenia	4.7
Ireland, Southern	4.4
Brazil, Sao Paulo	3.8
US, Los Angeles: Japanese	3.3
Japan, Miyagi	3.3
US, Puerto Rico	3.1
Singapore: Chinese	2.9
Hungary, Szabolcs-Szatmar	2.9
Hong Kong	2.8
Costa Rica	2.7
Singapore: Indian	2.6 *
Colombia, Cali	2.3
China, Shanghai	1.8
Romania, County Cluj	1.7
Kuwait: Kuwaitis	1.6
India, Bombay	1.5
Philippines, Rizal	1.5
Canada, Northwest Terr. & Yukon	15.0
India, Poona	0.7

Sweden	6.4
Denmark	6.2
France, Bas-Rhin	4.7
Norway	4.7
US, Connecticut: Black	4.5
FRG, Saarland	4.5
Switzerland, Geneva	4.5
German Democratic Republic	4.4
Australia, New South Wales	4.4
Netherlands, Eindhoven	4.3
US, Connecticut: White	4.2
Poland, Cracow City	4.2
Israel: All Jews	4.0
Canada	3.9
US, Los Angeles: Other White	3.7
US, Los Angeles: Black	3.6
UK, Scotland	3.4
Italy, Varese	3.1
Ireland, Southern	2.7
New Zealand: Maori	2.7
US, Los Angeles: Chinese	2.6 *
UK, England & Wales	2.5
Yugoslavia, Slovenia	2.5
Brazil, Sao Paulo	2.3
Hawaii: Hawaiian	2.3 *
Hungary, Szabolcs-Szatmar	2.2
Hong Kong	2.0
Spain, Navarra	1.9
Colombia, Cali	1.8
US, Los Angeles: Japanese	1.8 *
Costa Rica	1.7
Kuwait: Kuwaitis	1.7
US, Puerto Rico	1.6
Japan, Miyagi	1.6
Singapore: Chinese	1.5
Romania, County Cluj	1.3
Philippines, Rizal	1.1
China, Shanghai	1.0
India, Bombay	0.6
Singapore: Indian	0.4 *
Iceland	7.6
India, Poona	0.6

* Rates based on less than 10 cases

40

190 EYE

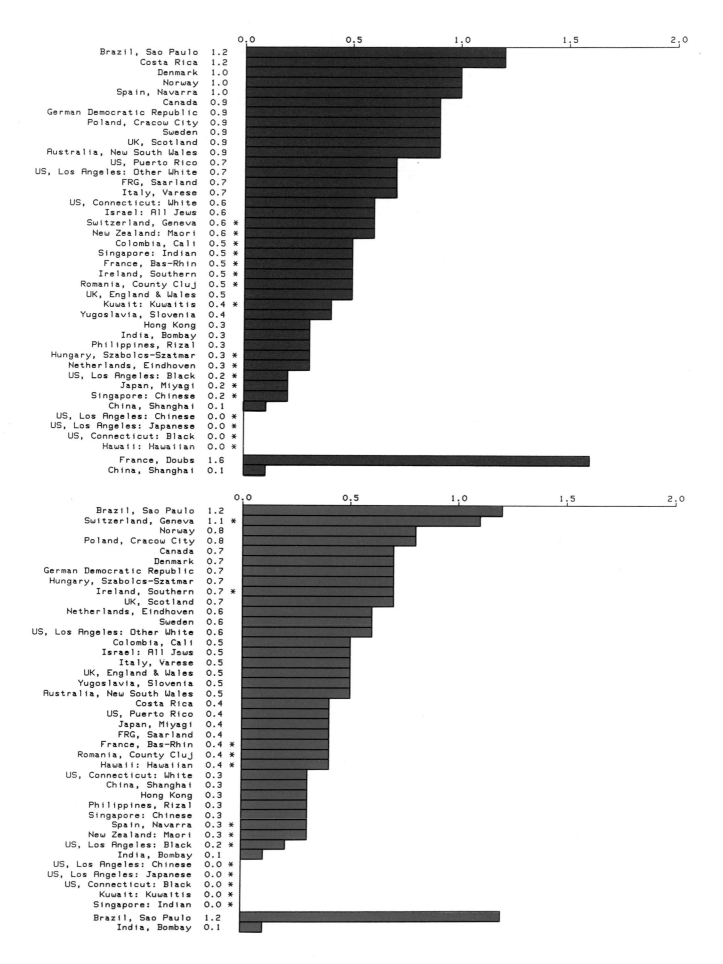

191-2 BRAIN, NERVOUS SYSTEM

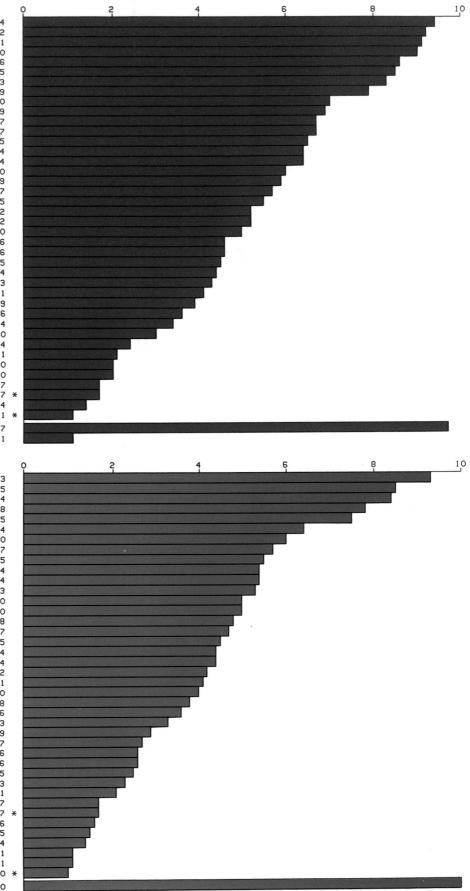

Sweden	9.4
US, Los Angeles: Other White	9.2
New Zealand: Maori	9.1
Israel: All Jews	9.0
Poland, Cracow City	8.6
Denmark	8.5
Norway	8.3
Spain, Navarra	7.9
Ireland, Southern	7.0
Brazil, Sao Paulo	6.9
Canada	6.7
US, Connecticut: White	6.7
Netherlands, Eindhoven	6.5
US, Los Angeles: Black	6.4
Australia, New South Wales	6.4
France, Bas-Rhin	6.0
UK, Scotland	5.9
FRG, Saarland	5.7
Italy, Varese	5.5
US, Los Angeles: Chinese	5.2
UK, England & Wales	5.2
German Democratic Republic	5.0
Colombia, Cali	4.6
US, Connecticut: Black	4.6
Switzerland, Geneva	4.5
Romania, County Cluj	4.4
US, Los Angeles: Japanese	4.3
Yugoslavia, Slovenia	4.1
Costa Rica	3.9
China, Shanghai	3.6
US, Puerto Rico	3.4
Hawaii: Hawaiian	3.0
Hungary, Szabolcs-Szatmar	2.4
India, Bombay	2.1
Hong Kong	2.0
Japan, Miyagi	2.0
Singapore: Chinese	1.7
Singapore: Indian	1.7 *
Philippines, Rizal	1.4
Kuwait: Kuwaitis	1.1 *
New Zealand: Pacific Polynesian	9.7
India, Nagpur	1.1

Sweden	9.3
Israel: All Jews	8.5
US, Los Angeles: Other White	8.4
Denmark	7.8
Norway	7.5
US, Los Angeles: Chinese	6.4
US, Los Angeles: Black	6.0
Spain, Navarra	5.7
Brazil, Sao Paulo	5.5
FRG, Saarland	5.4
Poland, Cracow City	5.4
Ireland, Southern	5.3
Canada	5.0
US, Connecticut: White	5.0
New Zealand: Maori	4.8
Australia, New South Wales	4.7
UK, Scotland	4.5
Italy, Varese	4.4
Switzerland, Geneva	4.4
German Democratic Republic	4.2
Hawaii: Hawaiian	4.1
France, Bas-Rhin	4.0
US, Los Angeles: Japanese	3.8
UK, England & Wales	3.6
Netherlands, Eindhoven	3.3
China, Shanghai	2.9
Romania, County Cluj	2.7
Colombia, Cali	2.6
Yugoslavia, Slovenia	2.6
US, Connecticut: Black	2.5
Costa Rica	2.3
US, Puerto Rico	2.1
Japan, Miyagi	1.7
Singapore: Indian	1.7 *
Hong Kong	1.6
India, Bombay	1.5
Hungary, Szabolcs-Szatmar	1.4
Philippines, Rizal	1.1
Singapore: Chinese	1.1
Kuwait: Kuwaitis	1.0 *
Iceland	10.0
India, Madras	0.8

* Rates based on less than 10 cases

42

193 THYROID

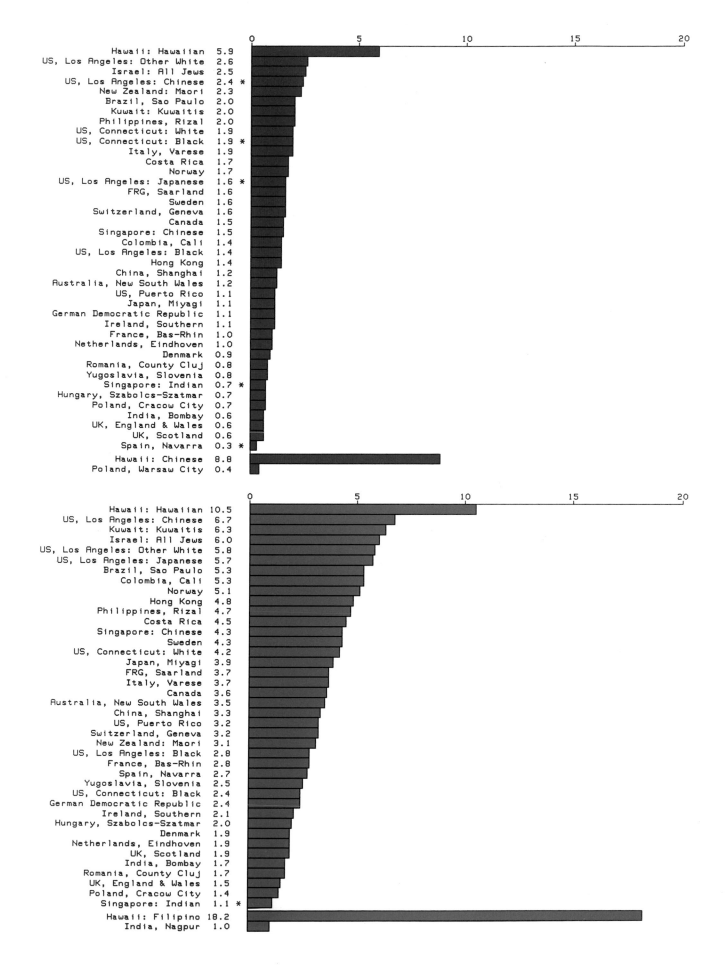

Hawaii: Hawaiian 5.9
US, Los Angeles: Other White 2.6
Israel: All Jews 2.5
US, Los Angeles: Chinese 2.4 *
New Zealand: Maori 2.3
Brazil, Sao Paulo 2.0
Kuwait: Kuwaitis 2.0
Philippines, Rizal 2.0
US, Connecticut: White 1.9
US, Connecticut: Black 1.9 *
Italy, Varese 1.9
Costa Rica 1.7
Norway 1.7
US, Los Angeles: Japanese 1.6 *
FRG, Saarland 1.6
Sweden 1.6
Switzerland, Geneva 1.6
Canada 1.5
Singapore: Chinese 1.5
Colombia, Cali 1.4
US, Los Angeles: Black 1.4
Hong Kong 1.4
China, Shanghai 1.2
Australia, New South Wales 1.2
US, Puerto Rico 1.1
Japan, Miyagi 1.1
German Democratic Republic 1.1
Ireland, Southern 1.1
France, Bas-Rhin 1.0
Netherlands, Eindhoven 1.0
Denmark 0.9
Romania, County Cluj 0.8
Yugoslavia, Slovenia 0.8
Singapore: Indian 0.7 *
Hungary, Szabolcs-Szatmar 0.7
Poland, Cracow City 0.7
India, Bombay 0.6
UK, England & Wales 0.6
UK, Scotland 0.6
Spain, Navarra 0.3 *

Hawaii: Chinese 8.8
Poland, Warsaw City 0.4

Hawaii: Hawaiian 10.5
US, Los Angeles: Chinese 6.7
Kuwait: Kuwaitis 6.3
Israel: All Jews 6.0
US, Los Angeles: Other White 5.8
US, Los Angeles: Japanese 5.7
Brazil, Sao Paulo 5.3
Colombia, Cali 5.3
Norway 5.1
Hong Kong 4.8
Philippines, Rizal 4.7
Costa Rica 4.5
Singapore: Chinese 4.3
Sweden 4.3
US, Connecticut: White 4.2
Japan, Miyagi 3.9
FRG, Saarland 3.7
Italy, Varese 3.7
Canada 3.6
Australia, New South Wales 3.5
China, Shanghai 3.3
US, Puerto Rico 3.2
Switzerland, Geneva 3.2
New Zealand: Maori 3.1
US, Los Angeles: Black 2.8
France, Bas-Rhin 2.8
Spain, Navarra 2.7
Yugoslavia, Slovenia 2.5
US, Connecticut: Black 2.4
German Democratic Republic 2.4
Ireland, Southern 2.1
Hungary, Szabolcs-Szatmar 2.0
Denmark 1.9
Netherlands, Eindhoven 1.9
UK, Scotland 1.9
India, Bombay 1.7
Romania, County Cluj 1.7
UK, England & Wales 1.5
Poland, Cracow City 1.4
Singapore: Indian 1.1 *

Hawaii: Filipino 18.2
India, Nagpur 1.0

* Rates based on less than 10 cases

194 OTHER ENDOCRINE

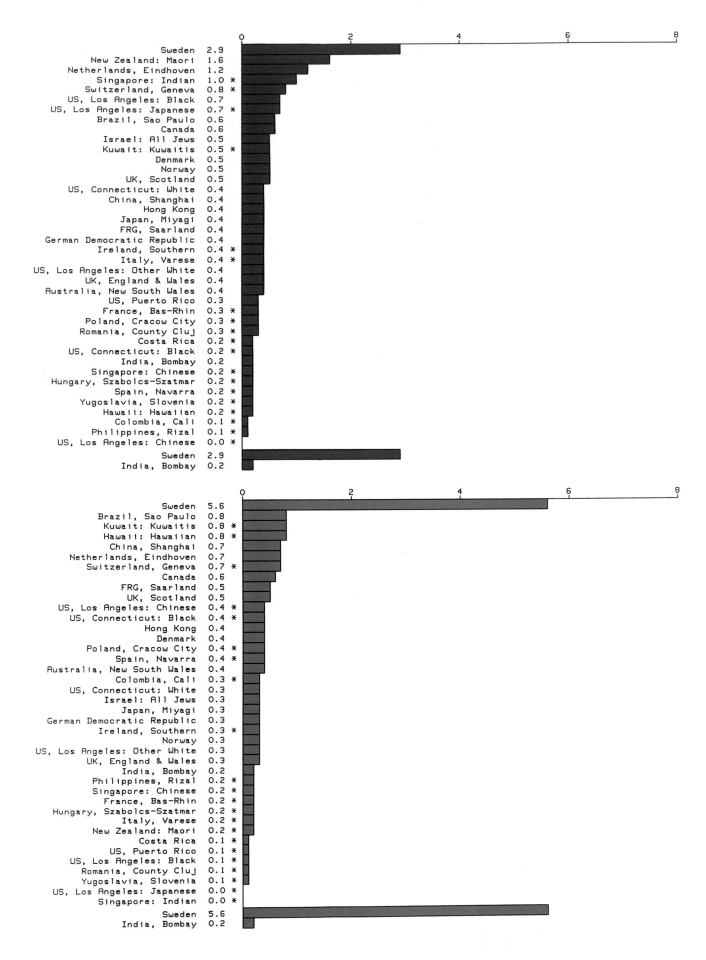

Sweden 2.9
New Zealand: Maori 1.6
Netherlands, Eindhoven 1.2
Singapore: Indian 1.0 *
Switzerland, Geneva 0.8 *
US, Los Angeles: Black 0.7
US, Los Angeles: Japanese 0.7 *
Brazil, Sao Paulo 0.6
Canada 0.6
Israel: All Jews 0.5
Kuwait: Kuwaitis 0.5 *
Denmark 0.5
Norway 0.5
UK, Scotland 0.5
US, Connecticut: White 0.4
China, Shanghai 0.4
Hong Kong 0.4
Japan, Miyagi 0.4
FRG, Saarland 0.4
German Democratic Republic 0.4
Ireland, Southern 0.4 *
Italy, Varese 0.4 *
US, Los Angeles: Other White 0.4
UK, England & Wales 0.4
Australia, New South Wales 0.4
US, Puerto Rico 0.3
France, Bas-Rhin 0.3 *
Poland, Cracow City 0.3 *
Romania, County Cluj 0.3 *
Costa Rica 0.2 *
US, Connecticut: Black 0.2 *
India, Bombay 0.2
Singapore: Chinese 0.2 *
Hungary, Szabolcs-Szatmar 0.2 *
Spain, Navarra 0.2 *
Yugoslavia, Slovenia 0.2 *
Hawaii: Hawaiian 0.2 *
Colombia, Cali 0.1 *
Philippines, Rizal 0.1 *
US, Los Angeles: Chinese 0.0 *
Sweden 2.9
India, Bombay 0.2

Sweden 5.6
Brazil, Sao Paulo 0.8
Kuwait: Kuwaitis 0.8 *
Hawaii: Hawaiian 0.8 *
China, Shanghai 0.7
Netherlands, Eindhoven 0.7
Switzerland, Geneva 0.7 *
Canada 0.6
FRG, Saarland 0.5
UK, Scotland 0.5
US, Los Angeles: Chinese 0.4 *
US, Connecticut: Black 0.4 *
Hong Kong 0.4
Denmark 0.4
Poland, Cracow City 0.4 *
Spain, Navarra 0.4 *
Australia, New South Wales 0.4
Colombia, Cali 0.3 *
US, Connecticut: White 0.3
Israel: All Jews 0.3
Japan, Miyagi 0.3
German Democratic Republic 0.3
Ireland, Southern 0.3 *
Norway 0.3
US, Los Angeles: Other White 0.3
UK, England & Wales 0.3
India, Bombay 0.2
Philippines, Rizal 0.2 *
Singapore: Chinese 0.2 *
France, Bas-Rhin 0.2 *
Hungary, Szabolcs-Szatmar 0.2 *
Italy, Varese 0.2 *
New Zealand: Maori 0.2 *
Costa Rica 0.1 *
US, Puerto Rico 0.1 *
US, Los Angeles: Black 0.1 *
Romania, County Cluj 0.1 *
Yugoslavia, Slovenia 0.1 *
US, Los Angeles: Japanese 0.0 *
Singapore: Indian 0.0 *
Sweden 5.6
India, Bombay 0.2

NOTE For Sweden, 194 includes all benign and malignant tumours

* Rates based on less than 10 cases

44

200 + 202 NON-HODGKIN LYMPHOMA

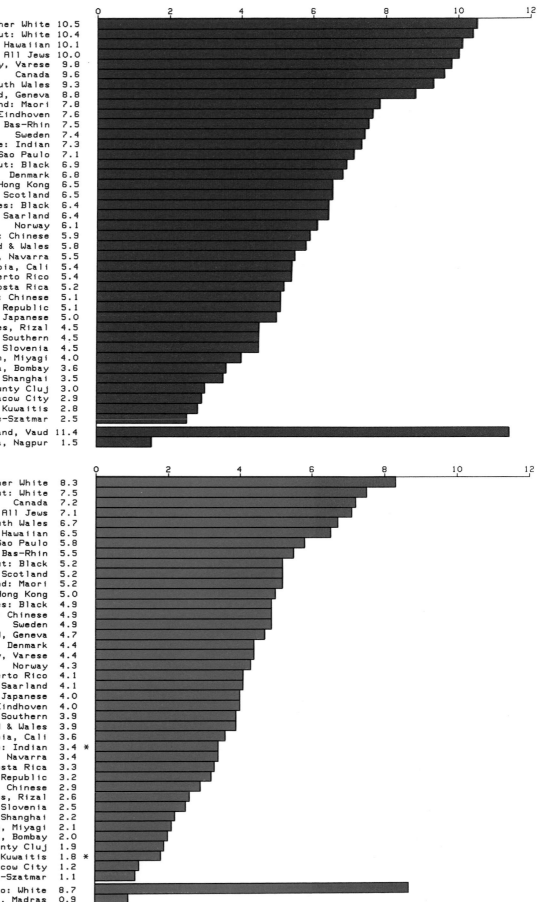

US, Los Angeles: Other White 10.5
US, Connecticut: White 10.4
Hawaii: Hawaiian 10.1
Israel: All Jews 10.0
Italy, Varese 9.8
Canada 9.6
Australia, New South Wales 9.3
Switzerland, Geneva 8.8
New Zealand: Maori 7.8
Netherlands, Eindhoven 7.6
France, Bas-Rhin 7.5
Sweden 7.4
Singapore: Indian 7.3
Brazil, Sao Paulo 7.1
US, Connecticut: Black 6.9
Denmark 6.8
Hong Kong 6.5
UK, Scotland 6.5
US, Los Angeles: Black 6.4
FRG, Saarland 6.4
Norway 6.1
US, Los Angeles: Chinese 5.9
UK, England & Wales 5.8
Spain, Navarra 5.5
Colombia, Cali 5.4
US, Puerto Rico 5.4
Costa Rica 5.2
Singapore: Chinese 5.1
German Democratic Republic 5.1
US, Los Angeles: Japanese 5.0
Philippines, Rizal 4.5
Ireland, Southern 4.5
Yugoslavia, Slovenia 4.5
Japan, Miyagi 4.0
India, Bombay 3.6
China, Shanghai 3.5
Romania, County Cluj 3.0
Poland, Cracow City 2.9
Kuwait: Kuwaitis 2.8
Hungary, Szabolcs-Szatmar 2.5

Switzerland, Vaud 11.4
India, Nagpur 1.5

US, Los Angeles: Other White 8.3
US, Connecticut: White 7.5
Canada 7.2
Israel: All Jews 7.1
Australia, New South Wales 6.7
Hawaii: Hawaiian 6.5
Brazil, Sao Paulo 5.8
France, Bas-Rhin 5.5
US, Connecticut: Black 5.2
UK, Scotland 5.2
New Zealand: Maori 5.2
Hong Kong 5.0
US, Los Angeles: Black 4.9
US, Los Angeles: Chinese 4.9
Sweden 4.9
Switzerland, Geneva 4.7
Denmark 4.4
Italy, Varese 4.4
Norway 4.3
US, Puerto Rico 4.1
FRG, Saarland 4.1
US, Los Angeles: Japanese 4.0
Netherlands, Eindhoven 4.0
Ireland, Southern 3.9
UK, England & Wales 3.9
Colombia, Cali 3.6
Singapore: Indian 3.4 *
Spain, Navarra 3.4
Costa Rica 3.3
German Democratic Republic 3.2
Singapore: Chinese 2.9
Philippines, Rizal 2.6
Yugoslavia, Slovenia 2.5
China, Shanghai 2.2
Japan, Miyagi 2.1
India, Bombay 2.0
Romania, County Cluj 1.9
Kuwait: Kuwaitis 1.8 *
Poland, Cracow City 1.2
Hungary, Szabolcs-Szatmar 1.1

US, San Francisco: White 8.7
India, Madras 0.9

* Rates based on less than 10 cases

45

201 HODGKIN'S DISEASE

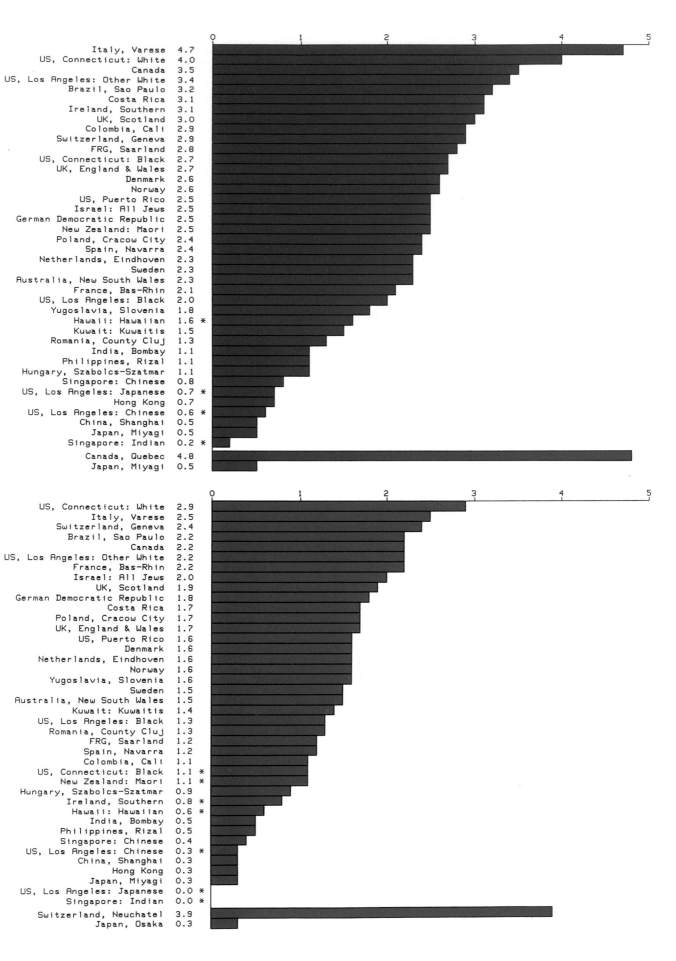

Italy, Varese	4.7
US, Connecticut: White	4.0
Canada	3.5
US, Los Angeles: Other White	3.4
Brazil, Sao Paulo	3.2
Costa Rica	3.1
Ireland, Southern	3.1
UK, Scotland	3.0
Colombia, Cali	2.9
Switzerland, Geneva	2.9
FRG, Saarland	2.8
US, Connecticut: Black	2.7
UK, England & Wales	2.7
Denmark	2.6
Norway	2.6
US, Puerto Rico	2.5
Israel: All Jews	2.5
German Democratic Republic	2.5
New Zealand: Maori	2.5
Poland, Cracow City	2.4
Spain, Navarra	2.4
Netherlands, Eindhoven	2.3
Sweden	2.3
Australia, New South Wales	2.3
France, Bas-Rhin	2.1
US, Los Angeles: Black	2.0
Yugoslavia, Slovenia	1.8
Hawaii: Hawaiian	1.6 *
Kuwait: Kuwaitis	1.5
Romania, County Cluj	1.3
India, Bombay	1.1
Philippines, Rizal	1.1
Hungary, Szabolcs-Szatmar	1.1
Singapore: Chinese	0.8
US, Los Angeles: Japanese	0.7 *
Hong Kong	0.7
US, Los Angeles: Chinese	0.6 *
China, Shanghai	0.5
Japan, Miyagi	0.5
Singapore: Indian	0.2 *
Canada, Quebec	4.8
Japan, Miyagi	0.5

US, Connecticut: White	2.9
Italy, Varese	2.5
Switzerland, Geneva	2.4
Brazil, Sao Paulo	2.2
Canada	2.2
US, Los Angeles: Other White	2.2
France, Bas-Rhin	2.2
Israel: All Jews	2.0
UK, Scotland	1.9
German Democratic Republic	1.8
Costa Rica	1.7
Poland, Cracow City	1.7
UK, England & Wales	1.7
US, Puerto Rico	1.6
Denmark	1.6
Netherlands, Eindhoven	1.6
Norway	1.6
Yugoslavia, Slovenia	1.6
Sweden	1.5
Australia, New South Wales	1.5
Kuwait: Kuwaitis	1.4
US, Los Angeles: Black	1.3
Romania, County Cluj	1.3
FRG, Saarland	1.2
Spain, Navarra	1.2
Colombia, Cali	1.1
US, Connecticut: Black	1.1 *
New Zealand: Maori	1.1 *
Hungary, Szabolcs-Szatmar	0.9
Ireland, Southern	0.8 *
Hawaii: Hawaiian	0.6 *
India, Bombay	0.5
Philippines, Rizal	0.5
Singapore: Chinese	0.4
US, Los Angeles: Chinese	0.3 *
China, Shanghai	0.3
Hong Kong	0.3
Japan, Miyagi	0.3
US, Los Angeles: Japanese	0.0 *
Singapore: Indian	0.0 *
Switzerland, Neuchatel	3.9
Japan, Osaka	0.3

* Rates based on less than 10 cases

203 MULTIPLE MYELOMA

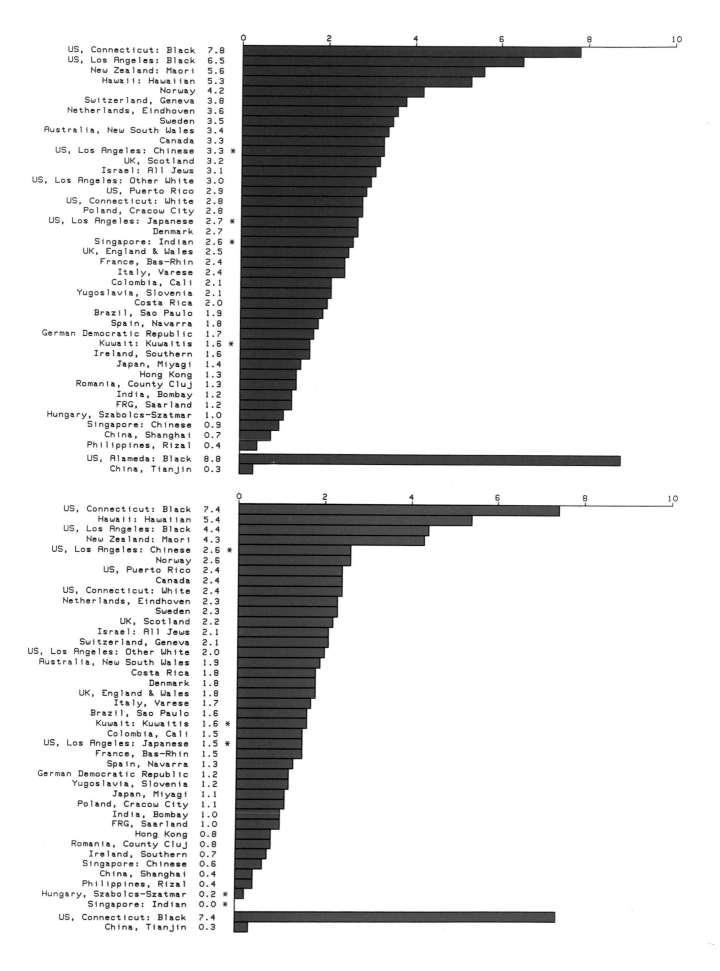

US, Connecticut: Black 7.8
US, Los Angeles: Black 6.5
New Zealand: Maori 5.6
Hawaii: Hawaiian 5.3
Norway 4.2
Switzerland, Geneva 3.8
Netherlands, Eindhoven 3.6
Sweden 3.5
Australia, New South Wales 3.4
Canada 3.3
US, Los Angeles: Chinese 3.3 *
UK, Scotland 3.2
Israel: All Jews 3.1
US, Los Angeles: Other White 3.0
US, Puerto Rico 2.9
US, Connecticut: White 2.8
Poland, Cracow City 2.8
US, Los Angeles: Japanese 2.7 *
Denmark 2.7
Singapore: Indian 2.6 *
UK, England & Wales 2.5
France, Bas-Rhin 2.4
Italy, Varese 2.4
Colombia, Cali 2.1
Yugoslavia, Slovenia 2.1
Costa Rica 2.0
Brazil, Sao Paulo 1.9
Spain, Navarra 1.8
German Democratic Republic 1.7
Kuwait: Kuwaitis 1.6 *
Ireland, Southern 1.6
Japan, Miyagi 1.4
Hong Kong 1.3
Romania, County Cluj 1.3
India, Bombay 1.2
FRG, Saarland 1.2
Hungary, Szabolcs-Szatmar 1.0
Singapore: Chinese 0.9
China, Shanghai 0.7
Philippines, Rizal 0.4
US, Alameda: Black 8.8
China, Tianjin 0.3

US, Connecticut: Black 7.4
Hawaii: Hawaiian 5.4
US, Los Angeles: Black 4.4
New Zealand: Maori 4.3
US, Los Angeles: Chinese 2.6 *
Norway 2.6
US, Puerto Rico 2.4
Canada 2.4
US, Connecticut: White 2.4
Netherlands, Eindhoven 2.3
Sweden 2.3
UK, Scotland 2.2
Israel: All Jews 2.1
Switzerland, Geneva 2.1
US, Los Angeles: Other White 2.0
Australia, New South Wales 1.9
Costa Rica 1.8
Denmark 1.8
UK, England & Wales 1.8
Italy, Varese 1.7
Brazil, Sao Paulo 1.6
Kuwait: Kuwaitis 1.6 *
Colombia, Cali 1.5
US, Los Angeles: Japanese 1.5 *
France, Bas-Rhin 1.5
Spain, Navarra 1.3
German Democratic Republic 1.2
Yugoslavia, Slovenia 1.2
Japan, Miyagi 1.1
Poland, Cracow City 1.1
India, Bombay 1.0
FRG, Saarland 1.0
Hong Kong 0.8
Romania, County Cluj 0.8
Ireland, Southern 0.7
Singapore: Chinese 0.6
China, Shanghai 0.4
Philippines, Rizal 0.4
Hungary, Szabolcs-Szatmar 0.2 *
Singapore: Indian 0.0 *
US, Connecticut: Black 7.4
China, Tianjin 0.3

* Rates based on less than 10 cases

47

204 LYMPHOID LEUKAEMIA

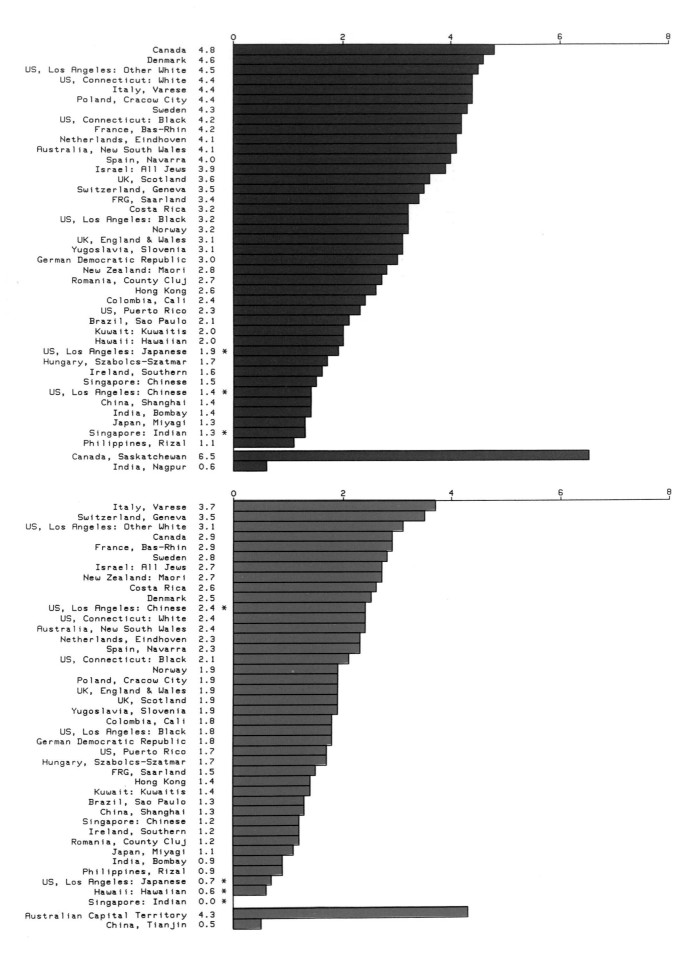

Canada	4.8
Denmark	4.6
US, Los Angeles: Other White	4.5
US, Connecticut: White	4.4
Italy, Varese	4.4
Poland, Cracow City	4.4
Sweden	4.3
US, Connecticut: Black	4.2
France, Bas-Rhin	4.2
Netherlands, Eindhoven	4.1
Australia, New South Wales	4.1
Spain, Navarra	4.0
Israel: All Jews	3.9
UK, Scotland	3.6
Switzerland, Geneva	3.5
FRG, Saarland	3.4
Costa Rica	3.2
US, Los Angeles: Black	3.2
Norway	3.2
UK, England & Wales	3.1
Yugoslavia, Slovenia	3.1
German Democratic Republic	3.0
New Zealand: Maori	2.8
Romania, County Cluj	2.7
Hong Kong	2.6
Colombia, Cali	2.4
US, Puerto Rico	2.3
Brazil, Sao Paulo	2.1
Kuwait: Kuwaitis	2.0
Hawaii: Hawaiian	2.0
US, Los Angeles: Japanese	1.9 *
Hungary, Szabolcs-Szatmar	1.7
Ireland, Southern	1.6
Singapore: Chinese	1.5
US, Los Angeles: Chinese	1.4 *
China, Shanghai	1.4
India, Bombay	1.4
Japan, Miyagi	1.3
Singapore: Indian	1.3 *
Philippines, Rizal	1.1
Canada, Saskatchewan	6.5
India, Nagpur	0.6

Italy, Varese	3.7
Switzerland, Geneva	3.5
US, Los Angeles: Other White	3.1
Canada	2.9
France, Bas-Rhin	2.9
Sweden	2.8
Israel: All Jews	2.7
New Zealand: Maori	2.7
Costa Rica	2.6
Denmark	2.5
US, Los Angeles: Chinese	2.4 *
US, Connecticut: White	2.4
Australia, New South Wales	2.4
Netherlands, Eindhoven	2.3
Spain, Navarra	2.3
US, Connecticut: Black	2.1
Norway	1.9
Poland, Cracow City	1.9
UK, England & Wales	1.9
UK, Scotland	1.9
Yugoslavia, Slovenia	1.9
Colombia, Cali	1.8
US, Los Angeles: Black	1.8
German Democratic Republic	1.8
US, Puerto Rico	1.7
Hungary, Szabolcs-Szatmar	1.7
FRG, Saarland	1.5
Hong Kong	1.4
Kuwait: Kuwaitis	1.4
Brazil, Sao Paulo	1.3
China, Shanghai	1.3
Singapore: Chinese	1.2
Ireland, Southern	1.2
Romania, County Cluj	1.2
Japan, Miyagi	1.1
India, Bombay	0.9
Philippines, Rizal	0.9
US, Los Angeles: Japanese	0.7 *
Hawaii: Hawaiian	0.6 *
Singapore: Indian	0.0 *
Australian Capital Territory	4.3
China, Tianjin	0.5

* Rates based on less than 10 cases

205 MYELOID LEUKAEMIA

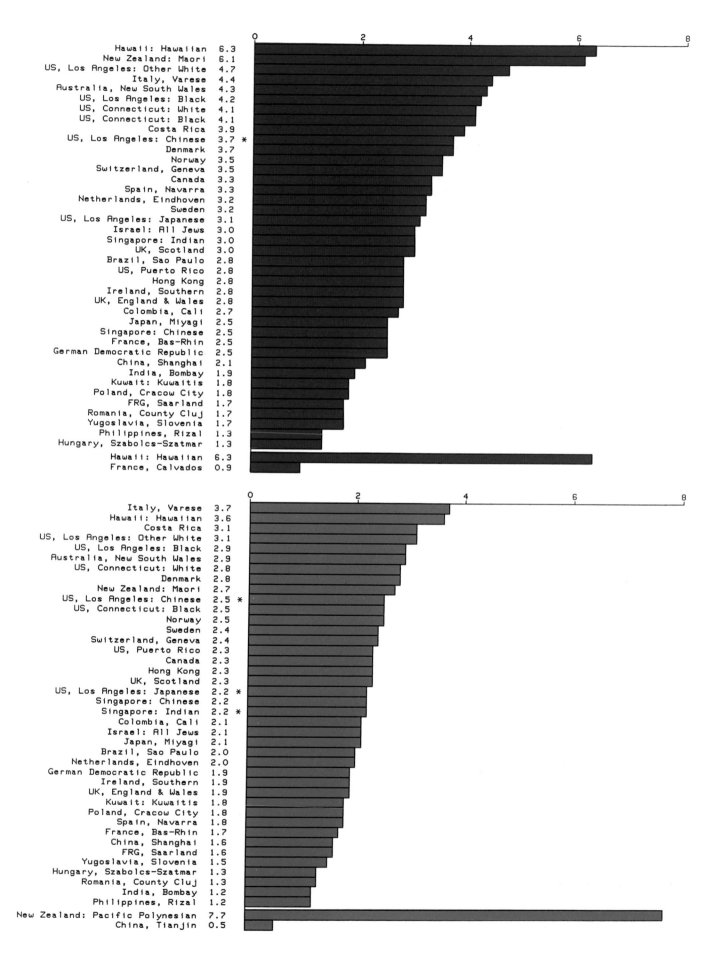

Hawaii: Hawaiian	6.3
New Zealand: Maori	6.1
US, Los Angeles: Other White	4.7
Italy, Varese	4.4
Australia, New South Wales	4.3
US, Los Angeles: Black	4.2
US, Connecticut: White	4.1
US, Connecticut: Black	4.1
Costa Rica	3.9
US, Los Angeles: Chinese	3.7 *
Denmark	3.7
Norway	3.5
Switzerland, Geneva	3.5
Canada	3.3
Spain, Navarra	3.3
Netherlands, Eindhoven	3.2
Sweden	3.2
US, Los Angeles: Japanese	3.1
Israel: All Jews	3.0
Singapore: Indian	3.0
UK, Scotland	3.0
Brazil, Sao Paulo	2.8
US, Puerto Rico	2.8
Hong Kong	2.8
Ireland, Southern	2.8
UK, England & Wales	2.8
Colombia, Cali	2.7
Japan, Miyagi	2.5
Singapore: Chinese	2.5
France, Bas-Rhin	2.5
German Democratic Republic	2.5
China, Shanghai	2.1
India, Bombay	1.9
Kuwait: Kuwaitis	1.8
Poland, Cracow City	1.8
FRG, Saarland	1.7
Romania, County Cluj	1.7
Yugoslavia, Slovenia	1.7
Philippines, Rizal	1.3
Hungary, Szabolcs-Szatmar	1.3
Hawaii: Hawaiian	6.3
France, Calvados	0.9

Italy, Varese	3.7
Hawaii: Hawaiian	3.6
Costa Rica	3.1
US, Los Angeles: Other White	3.1
US, Los Angeles: Black	2.9
Australia, New South Wales	2.9
US, Connecticut: White	2.8
Denmark	2.8
New Zealand: Maori	2.7
US, Los Angeles: Chinese	2.5 *
US, Connecticut: Black	2.5
Norway	2.5
Sweden	2.4
Switzerland, Geneva	2.4
US, Puerto Rico	2.3
Canada	2.3
Hong Kong	2.3
UK, Scotland	2.3
US, Los Angeles: Japanese	2.2 *
Singapore: Chinese	2.2
Singapore: Indian	2.2 *
Colombia, Cali	2.1
Israel: All Jews	2.1
Japan, Miyagi	2.1
Brazil, Sao Paulo	2.0
Netherlands, Eindhoven	2.0
German Democratic Republic	1.9
Ireland, Southern	1.9
UK, England & Wales	1.9
Kuwait: Kuwaitis	1.8
Poland, Cracow City	1.8
Spain, Navarra	1.8
France, Bas-Rhin	1.7
China, Shanghai	1.6
FRG, Saarland	1.6
Yugoslavia, Slovenia	1.5
Hungary, Szabolcs-Szatmar	1.3
Romania, County Cluj	1.3
India, Bombay	1.2
Philippines, Rizal	1.2
New Zealand: Pacific Polynesian	7.7
China, Tianjin	0.5

* Rates based on less than 10 cases

49

206 MONOCYTIC LEUKAEMIA

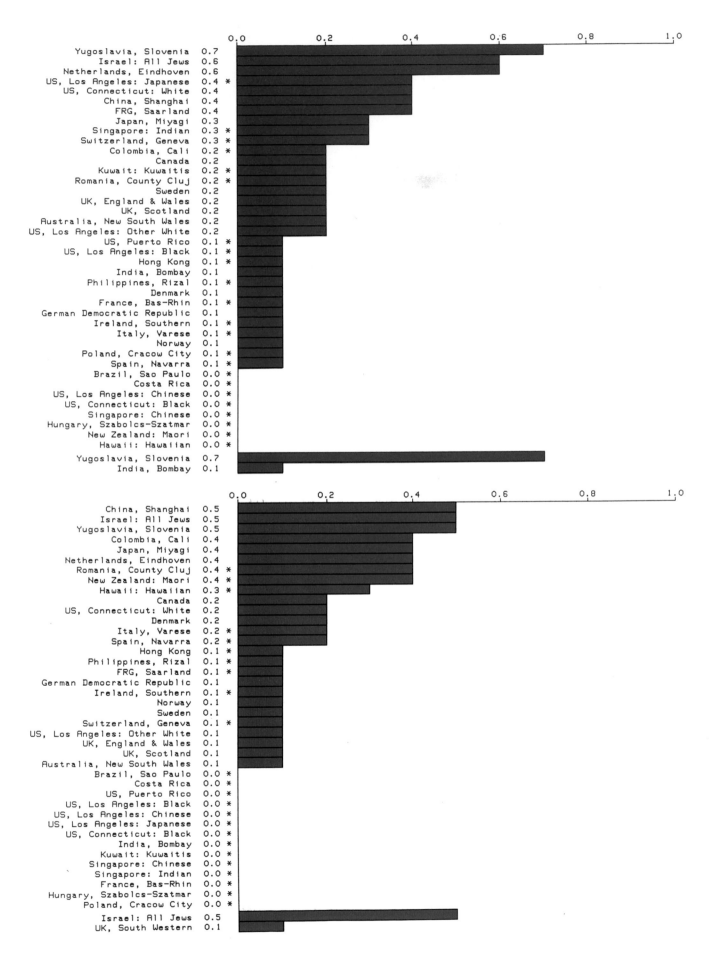

207 OTHER LEUKAEMIA

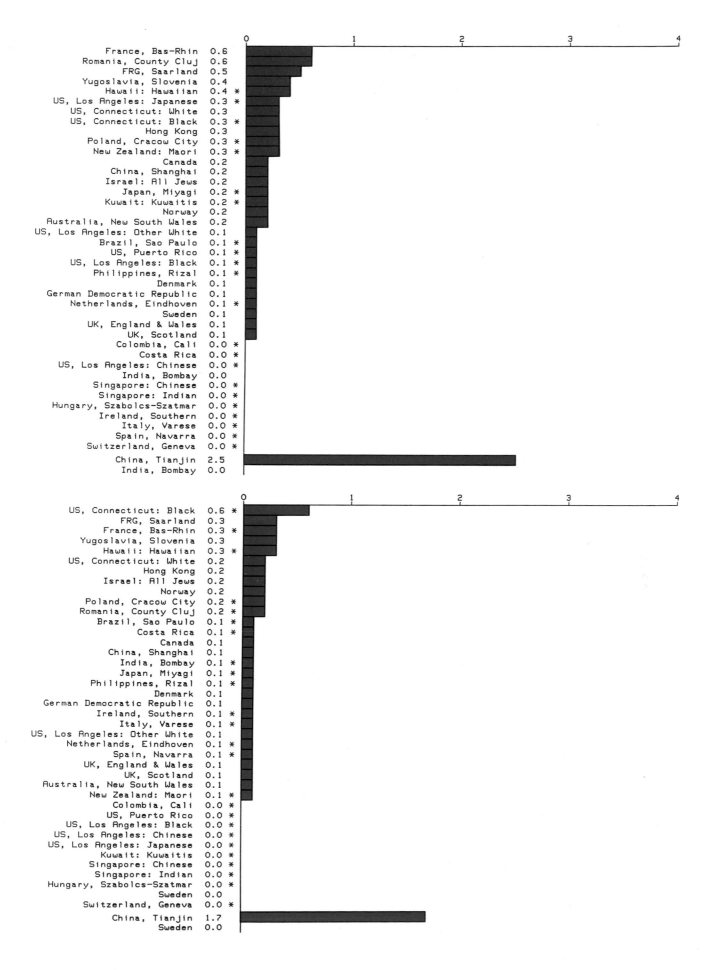

* Rates based on less than 10 cases

208 LEUKAEMIA, CELL UNSPECIFIED

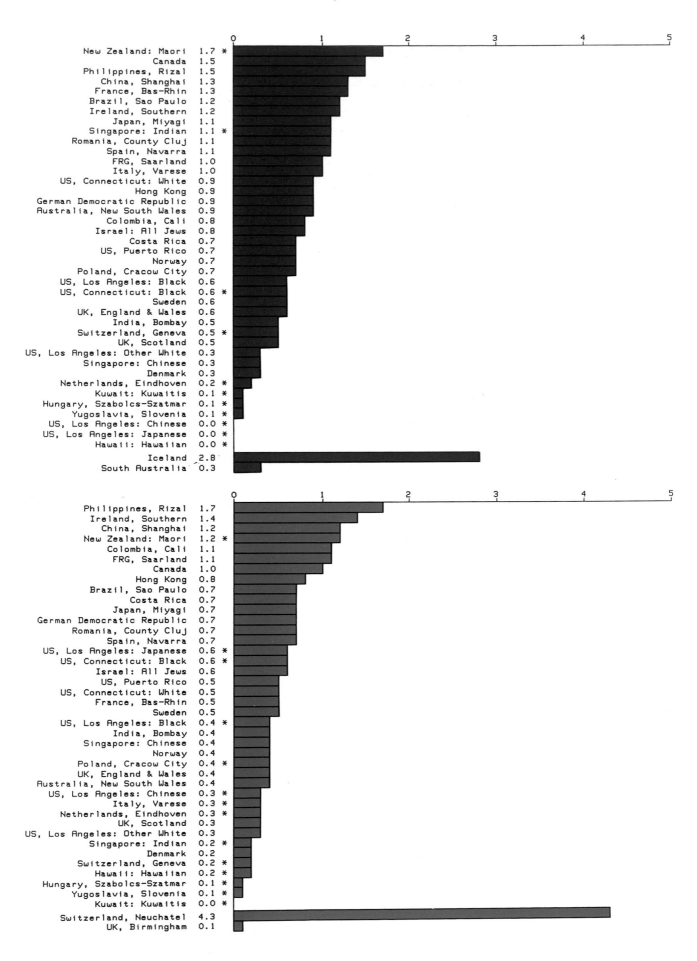

New Zealand: Maori 1.7 *
Canada 1.5
Philippines, Rizal 1.5
China, Shanghai 1.3
France, Bas-Rhin 1.3
Brazil, Sao Paulo 1.2
Ireland, Southern 1.2
Japan, Miyagi 1.1
Singapore: Indian 1.1 *
Romania, County Cluj 1.1
Spain, Navarra 1.1
FRG, Saarland 1.0
Italy, Varese 1.0
US, Connecticut: White 0.9
Hong Kong 0.9
German Democratic Republic 0.9
Australia, New South Wales 0.9
Colombia, Cali 0.8
Israel: All Jews 0.8
Costa Rica 0.7
US, Puerto Rico 0.7
Norway 0.7
Poland, Cracow City 0.7
US, Los Angeles: Black 0.6
US, Connecticut: Black 0.6 *
Sweden 0.6
UK, England & Wales 0.6
India, Bombay 0.5
Switzerland, Geneva 0.5 *
UK, Scotland 0.5
US, Los Angeles: Other White 0.3
Singapore: Chinese 0.3
Denmark 0.3
Netherlands, Eindhoven 0.2 *
Kuwait: Kuwaitis 0.1 *
Hungary, Szabolcs-Szatmar 0.1 *
Yugoslavia, Slovenia 0.1 *
US, Los Angeles: Chinese 0.0 *
US, Los Angeles: Japanese 0.0 *
Hawaii: Hawaiian 0.0 *
Iceland 2.8
South Australia 0.3

Philippines, Rizal 1.7
Ireland, Southern 1.4
China, Shanghai 1.2
New Zealand: Maori 1.2 *
Colombia, Cali 1.1
FRG, Saarland 1.1
Canada 1.0
Hong Kong 0.8
Brazil, Sao Paulo 0.7
Costa Rica 0.7
Japan, Miyagi 0.7
German Democratic Republic 0.7
Romania, County Cluj 0.7
Spain, Navarra 0.7
US, Los Angeles: Japanese 0.6 *
US, Connecticut: Black 0.6 *
Israel: All Jews 0.6
US, Puerto Rico 0.5
US, Connecticut: White 0.5
France, Bas-Rhin 0.5
Sweden 0.5
US, Los Angeles: Black 0.4 *
India, Bombay 0.4
Singapore: Chinese 0.4
Norway 0.4
Poland, Cracow City 0.4 *
UK, England & Wales 0.4
Australia, New South Wales 0.4
US, Los Angeles: Chinese 0.3 *
Italy, Varese 0.3 *
Netherlands, Eindhoven 0.3 *
UK, Scotland 0.3
US, Los Angeles: Other White 0.3
Singapore: Indian 0.2 *
Denmark 0.2
Switzerland, Geneva 0.2 *
Hawaii: Hawaiian 0.2 *
Hungary, Szabolcs-Szatmar 0.1 *
Yugoslavia, Slovenia 0.1 *
Kuwait: Kuwaitis 0.0 *
Switzerland, Neuchatel 4.3
UK, Birmingham 0.1

* Rates based on less than 10 cases

52

PRIMARY SITE UNCERTAIN

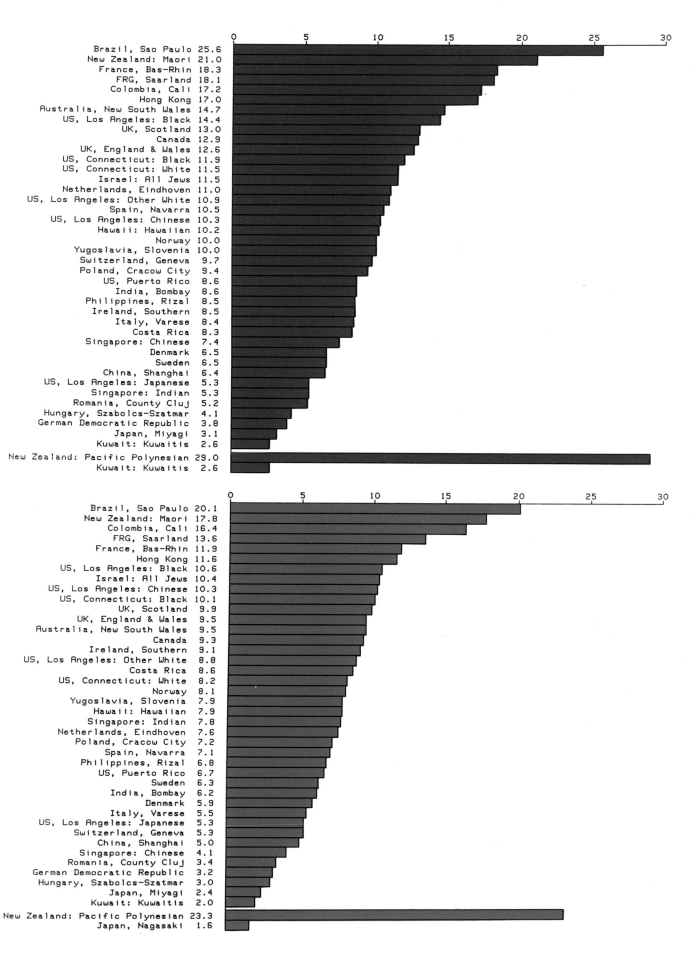

Brazil, Sao Paulo 25.6
New Zealand: Maori 21.0
France, Bas-Rhin 18.3
FRG, Saarland 18.1
Colombia, Cali 17.2
Hong Kong 17.0
Australia, New South Wales 14.7
US, Los Angeles: Black 14.4
UK, Scotland 13.0
Canada 12.9
UK, England & Wales 12.6
US, Connecticut: Black 11.9
US, Connecticut: White 11.5
Israel: All Jews 11.5
Netherlands, Eindhoven 11.0
US, Los Angeles: Other White 10.9
Spain, Navarra 10.5
US, Los Angeles: Chinese 10.3
Hawaii: Hawaiian 10.2
Norway 10.0
Yugoslavia, Slovenia 10.0
Switzerland, Geneva 9.7
Poland, Cracow City 9.4
US, Puerto Rico 8.6
India, Bombay 8.6
Philippines, Rizal 8.5
Ireland, Southern 8.5
Italy, Varese 8.4
Costa Rica 8.3
Singapore: Chinese 7.4
Denmark 6.5
Sweden 6.5
China, Shanghai 6.4
US, Los Angeles: Japanese 5.3
Singapore: Indian 5.3
Romania, County Cluj 5.2
Hungary, Szabolcs-Szatmar 4.1
German Democratic Republic 3.8
Japan, Miyagi 3.1
Kuwait: Kuwaitis 2.6

New Zealand: Pacific Polynesian 29.0
Kuwait: Kuwaitis 2.6

Brazil, Sao Paulo 20.1
New Zealand: Maori 17.8
Colombia, Cali 16.4
FRG, Saarland 13.6
France, Bas-Rhin 11.9
Hong Kong 11.6
US, Los Angeles: Black 10.6
Israel: All Jews 10.4
US, Los Angeles: Chinese 10.3
US, Connecticut: Black 10.1
UK, Scotland 9.9
UK, England & Wales 9.5
Australia, New South Wales 9.5
Canada 9.3
Ireland, Southern 9.1
US, Los Angeles: Other White 8.8
Costa Rica 8.6
US, Connecticut: White 8.2
Norway 8.1
Yugoslavia, Slovenia 7.9
Hawaii: Hawaiian 7.9
Singapore: Indian 7.8
Netherlands, Eindhoven 7.6
Poland, Cracow City 7.2
Spain, Navarra 7.1
Philippines, Rizal 6.8
US, Puerto Rico 6.7
Sweden 6.3
India, Bombay 6.2
Denmark 5.9
Italy, Varese 5.5
US, Los Angeles: Japanese 5.3
Switzerland, Geneva 5.3
China, Shanghai 5.0
Singapore: Chinese 4.1
Romania, County Cluj 3.4
German Democratic Republic 3.2
Hungary, Szabolcs-Szatmar 3.0
Japan, Miyagi 2.4
Kuwait: Kuwaitis 2.0

New Zealand: Pacific Polynesian 23.3
Japan, Nagasaki 1.6

ALL SITES BUT 173

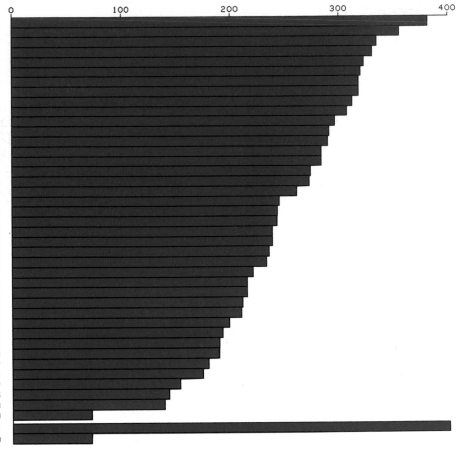

US, Connecticut: Black	381.5
US, Los Angeles: Black	355.2
Italy, Varese	334.5
France, Bas-Rhin	330.7
New Zealand: Maori	322.9
Switzerland, Geneva	319.9
Brazil, Sao Paulo	318.2
US, Connecticut: White	318.1
Hawaii: Hawaiian	311.9
US, Los Angeles: Other White	307.2
FRG, Saarland	296.3
Netherlands, Eindhoven	290.6
Canada	289.5
Hong Kong	283.7
UK, Scotland	283.7
Singapore: Chinese	273.6
Australia, New South Wales	272.8
Denmark	260.7
China, Shanghai	244.7
Spain, Navarra	243.0
Poland, Cracow City	242.6
UK, England & Wales	238.5
Norway	238.3
Yugoslavia, Slovenia	235.0
Sweden	233.2
German Democratic Republic	220.7
Israel: All Jews	215.3
Japan, Miyagi	215.1
US, Los Angeles: Chinese	211.2
Colombia, Cali	209.9
Costa Rica	198.5
Ireland, Southern	192.4
US, Puerto Rico	189.9
Hungary, Szabolcs-Szatmar	188.9
US, Los Angeles: Japanese	179.7
Romania, County Cluj	174.4
Singapore: Indian	153.7
India, Bombay	143.5
Philippines, Rizal	139.3
Kuwait: Kuwaitis	71.9
US, Detroit: Black	400.1
Kuwait: Kuwaitis	71.9

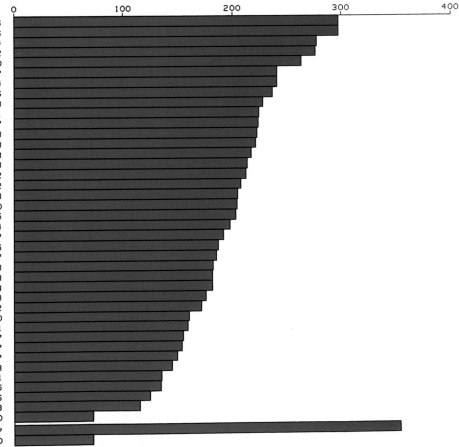

New Zealand: Maori	297.6
Hawaii: Hawaiian	297.6
Brazil, Sao Paulo	277.4
US, Los Angeles: Other White	276.2
US, Connecticut: White	263.0
Denmark	240.7
US, Connecticut: Black	240.4
Canada	236.6
US, Los Angeles: Black	227.3
Sweden	224.1
UK, Scotland	223.7
Switzerland, Geneva	222.3
Colombia, Cali	220.8
Israel: All Jews	216.8
FRG, Saarland	213.3
Norway	212.2
Australia, New South Wales	207.2
Italy, Varese	204.3
Netherlands, Eindhoven	204.0
France, Bas-Rhin	202.5
Hong Kong	197.4
UK, England & Wales	191.7
US, Los Angeles: Chinese	186.5
German Democratic Republic	184.7
Poland, Cracow City	182.3
Costa Rica	181.3
Ireland, Southern	181.3
Singapore: Chinese	175.3
Singapore: Indian	171.2
US, Los Angeles: Japanese	160.0
Yugoslavia, Slovenia	159.1
China, Shanghai	154.7
Spain, Navarra	153.7
US, Puerto Rico	149.7
Japan, Miyagi	144.8
Philippines, Rizal	135.1
Romania, County Cluj	134.5
India, Bombay	124.6
Hungary, Szabolcs-Szatmar	115.3
Kuwait: Kuwaitis	72.0
New Zealand: Pacific Polynesian	353.7
Kuwait: Kuwaitis	72.0

54

Part II

Pie diagrams showing relative frequencies of the ten top-ranking cancer sites

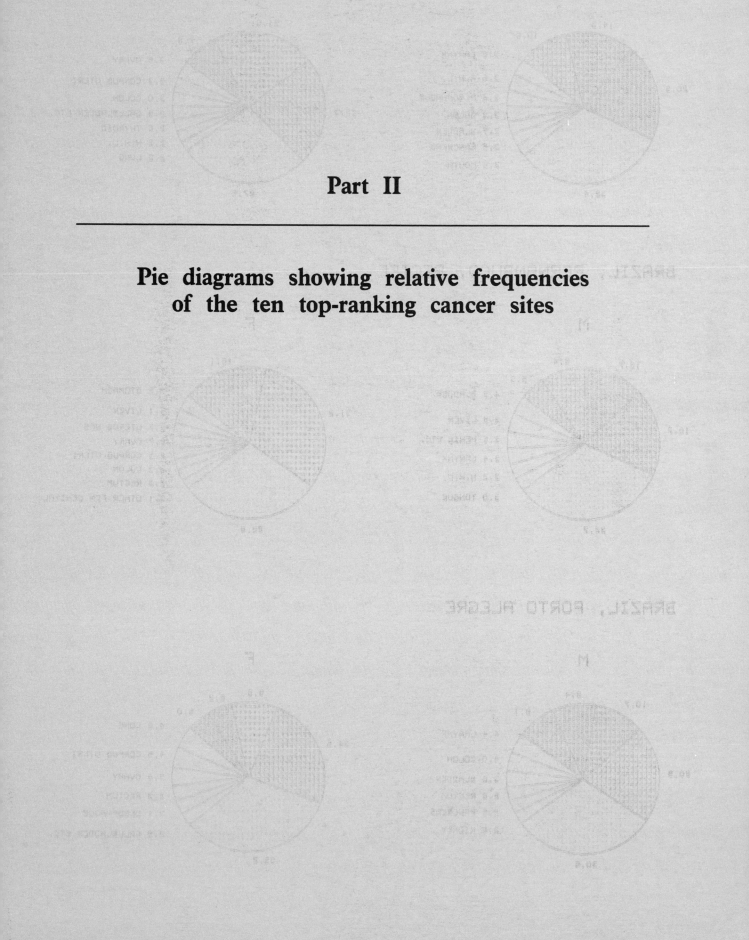

BRAZIL, FORTALEZA

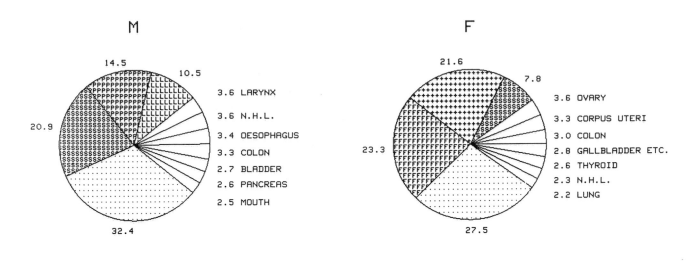

M

14.5
10.5
20.9
32.4

3.6 LARYNX
3.6 N.H.L.
3.4 OESOPHAGUS
3.3 COLON
2.7 BLADDER
2.6 PANCREAS
2.5 MOUTH

F

21.6
7.8
23.3
27.5

3.6 OVARY
3.3 CORPUS UTERI
3.0 COLON
2.8 GALLBLADDER ETC.
2.6 THYROID
2.3 N.H.L.
2.2 LUNG

BRAZIL, PERNAMBUCO, RECIFE

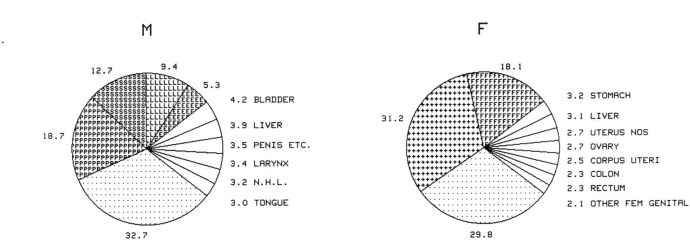

M

12.7
9.4
5.3
18.7
32.7

4.2 BLADDER
3.9 LIVER
3.5 PENIS ETC.
3.4 LARYNX
3.2 N.H.L.
3.0 TONGUE

F

18.1
31.2
29.8

3.2 STOMACH
3.1 LIVER
2.7 UTERUS NOS
2.7 OVARY
2.5 CORPUS UTERI
2.3 COLON
2.3 RECTUM
2.1 OTHER FEM GENITAL

BRAZIL, PORTO ALEGRE

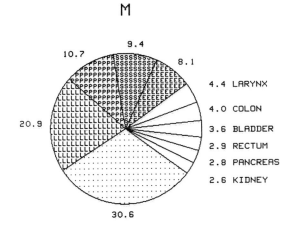

M

10.7
9.4
8.1
20.9
30.6

4.4 LARYNX
4.0 COLON
3.6 BLADDER
2.9 RECTUM
2.8 PANCREAS
2.6 KIDNEY

F

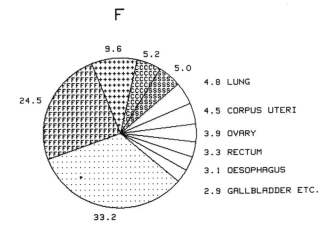

9.6
5.2
5.0
24.5
33.2

4.8 LUNG
4.5 CORPUS UTERI
3.9 OVARY
3.3 RECTUM
3.1 OESOPHAGUS
2.9 GALLBLADDER ETC.

BRAZIL, SAO PAULO

M

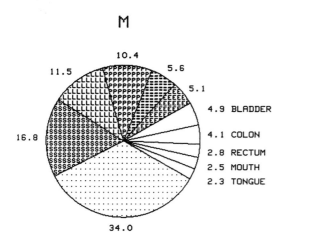

10.4
11.5
5.6
5.1
4.9 BLADDER
4.1 COLON
2.8 RECTUM
2.5 MOUTH
2.3 TONGUE
16.8
34.0

F

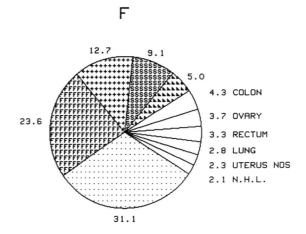

12.7
9.1
5.0
4.3 COLON
3.7 OVARY
3.3 RECTUM
2.8 LUNG
2.3 UTERUS NOS
2.1 N.H.L.
23.6
31.1

COLOMBIA, CALI

M

14.6
12.1
4.6 BLADDER
2.6 LARYNX
2.6 N.H.L.
2.5 COLON
2.5 PANCREAS
2.2 NERVOUS SYSTEM
1.6 RECTUM
23.6
31.1

F

15.8
11.9
4.4 LUNG
4.2 GALLBLADDER ETC.
3.5 OVARY
2.8 COLON
2.7 CORPUS UTERI
2.4 THYROID
1.7 RECTUM
21.8
28.8

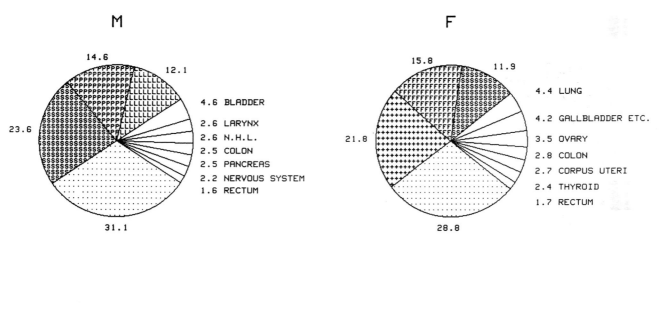

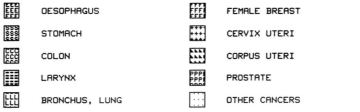

OESOPHAGUS	FEMALE BREAST	
STOMACH	CERVIX UTERI	
COLON	CORPUS UTERI	
LARYNX	PROSTATE	
BRONCHUS, LUNG	OTHER CANCERS	

COSTA RICA

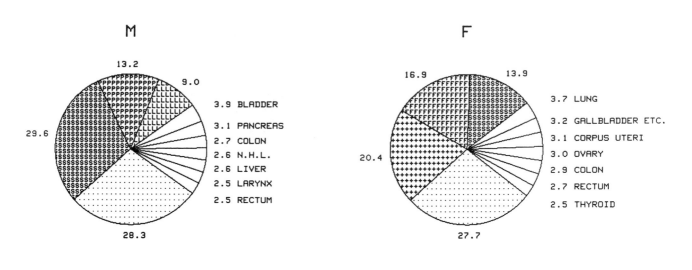

M

13.2
9.0
29.6
28.3

3.9 BLADDER
3.1 PANCREAS
2.7 COLON
2.6 N.H.L.
2.6 LIVER
2.5 LARYNX
2.5 RECTUM

F

16.9
13.9
20.4
27.7

3.7 LUNG
3.2 GALLBLADDER ETC.
3.1 CORPUS UTERI
3.0 OVARY
2.9 COLON
2.7 RECTUM
2.5 THYROID

FRANCE, MARTINIQUE

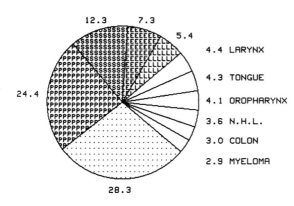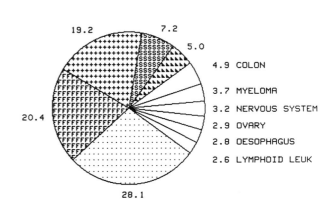

M

12.3   7.3
5.4
24.4
28.3

4.4 LARYNX
4.3 TONGUE
4.1 OROPHARYNX
3.6 N.H.L.
3.0 COLON
2.9 MYELOMA

F

19.2   7.2
5.0
20.4
28.1

4.9 COLON
3.7 MYELOMA
3.2 NERVOUS SYSTEM
2.9 OVARY
2.8 OESOPHAGUS
2.6 LYMPHOID LEUK

NETHERLANDS ANTILLES (LESS ARUBA)

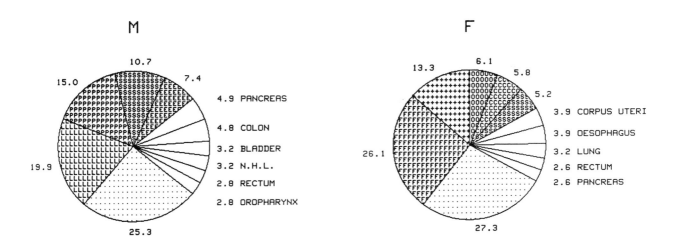

M

10.7
15.0   7.4
19.9
25.3

4.9 PANCREAS
4.8 COLON
3.2 BLADDER
3.2 N.H.L.
2.8 RECTUM
2.8 OROPHARYNX

F

13.3   6.1   5.8
5.2
26.1
27.3

3.9 CORPUS UTERI
3.9 OESOPHAGUS
3.2 LUNG
2.6 RECTUM
2.6 PANCREAS

USA, PUERTO RICO

M

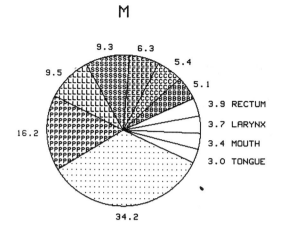

9.3   6.3
9.5   5.4
                5.1
16.2
        3.9 RECTUM
        3.7 LARYNX
        3.4 MOUTH
        3.0 TONGUE
        34.2

F

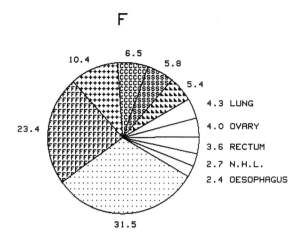

10.4   6.5
            5.8
                5.4
23.4
        4.3 LUNG
        4.0 OVARY
        3.6 RECTUM
        2.7 N.H.L.
        2.4 OESOPHAGUS
        31.5

CANADA

M

8.3
15.1   7.0
                5.3
21.2
        4.6 STOMACH
        3.3 N.H.L.
        3.0 PANCREAS
        2.7 KIDNEY
        2.4 LARYNX
        27.1

F

9.5   7.1
            7.1
28.1
        4.9 OVARY
        4.4 CERVIX UTERI
        4.1 RECTUM
        3.0 N.H.L.
        2.5 MELANOMA
        2.5 STOMACH
        26.8

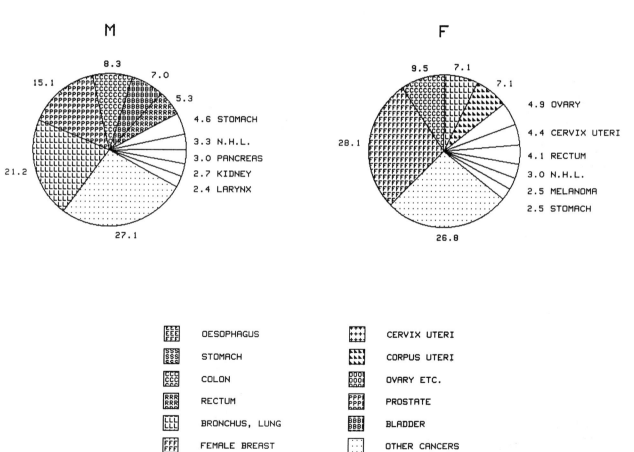

OESOPHAGUS		CERVIX UTERI
STOMACH		CORPUS UTERI
COLON		OVARY ETC.
RECTUM		PROSTATE
BRONCHUS, LUNG		BLADDER
FEMALE BREAST		OTHER CANCERS

CANADA, ALBERTA

M

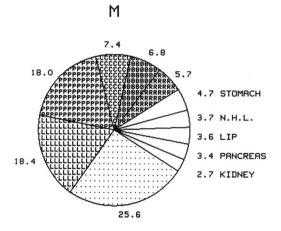

7.4
6.8
18.0
5.7
4.7 STOMACH
3.7 N.H.L.
3.6 LIP
3.4 PANCREAS
2.7 KIDNEY
18.4
25.6

F

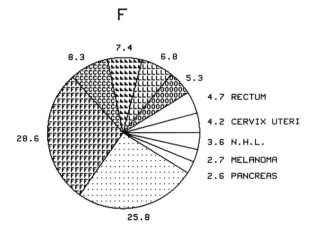

8.3
7.4
6.8
5.3
4.7 RECTUM
4.2 CERVIX UTERI
3.6 N.H.L.
2.7 MELANOMA
2.6 PANCREAS
28.6
25.8

CANADA, BRITISH COLUMBIA

M

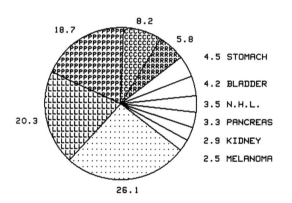

8.2
18.7
5.8
4.5 STOMACH
4.2 BLADDER
3.5 N.H.L.
3.3 PANCREAS
2.9 KIDNEY
2.5 MELANOMA
20.3
26.1

F

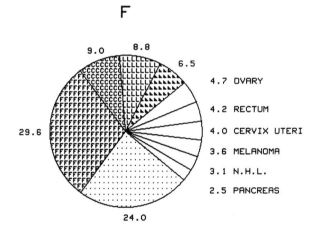

9.0
8.8
6.5
4.7 OVARY
4.2 RECTUM
4.0 CERVIX UTERI
3.6 MELANOMA
3.1 N.H.L.
2.5 PANCREAS
29.6
24.0

CANADA, MANITOBA

M

9.2
6.1
15.2
5.4
4.8 STOMACH
3.7 LIP
3.6 N.H.L.
3.2 KIDNEY
3.0 PANCREAS
21.1
24.7

F

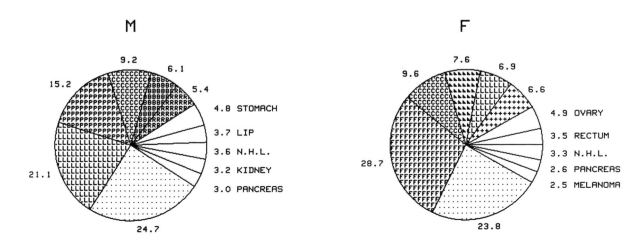

7.6
6.9
9.6
6.6
4.9 OVARY
3.5 RECTUM
3.3 N.H.L.
2.6 PANCREAS
2.5 MELANOMA
28.7
23.8

CANADA, MARITIME PROVINCES

M

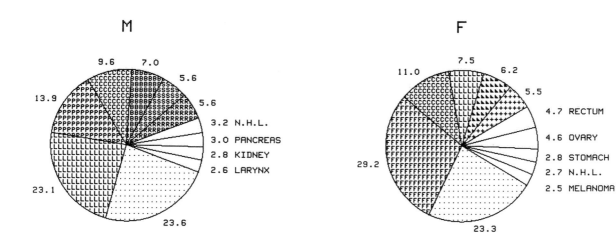

9.6   7.0
5.6
13.9
5.6
3.2 N.H.L.
3.0 PANCREAS
2.8 KIDNEY
2.6 LARYNX
23.1
23.6

F

7.5   6.2
11.0
5.5
4.7 RECTUM
4.6 OVARY
2.8 STOMACH
2.7 N.H.L.
2.5 MELANOMA
29.2
23.3

CANADA, NEW BRUNSWICK

M

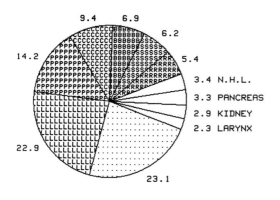

9.4   6.9
6.2
14.2
5.4
3.4 N.H.L.
3.3 PANCREAS
2.9 KIDNEY
2.3 LARYNX
22.9
23.1

F

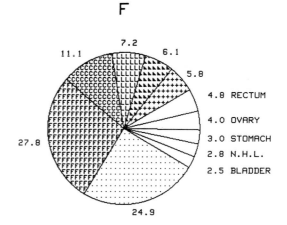

7.2   6.1
11.1
5.8
4.8 RECTUM
4.0 OVARY
3.0 STOMACH
2.8 N.H.L.
2.5 BLADDER
27.8
24.9

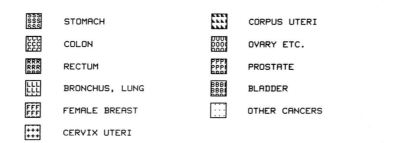

STOMACH	CORPUS UTERI
COLON	OVARY ETC.
RECTUM	PROSTATE
BRONCHUS, LUNG	BLADDER
FEMALE BREAST	OTHER CANCERS
CERVIX UTERI	

CANADA, NOVA SCOTIA

M

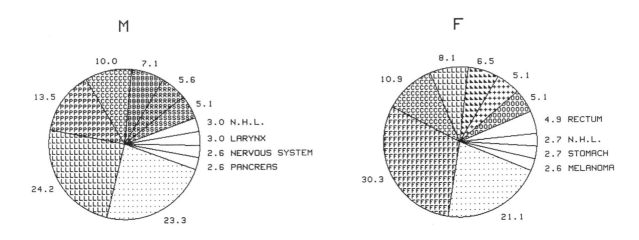

10.0   7.1
5.6
13.5
5.1
3.0 N.H.L.
3.0 LARYNX
2.6 NERVOUS SYSTEM
2.6 PANCREAS
24.2
23.3

F

8.1   6.5
5.1
10.9
5.1
4.9 RECTUM
2.7 N.H.L.
2.7 STOMACH
2.6 MELANOMA
30.3
21.1

CANADA, PRINCE EDWARD ISLAND

M

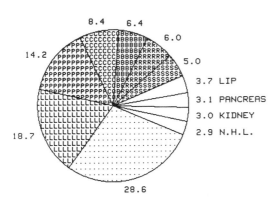

8.4   6.4
6.0
14.2
5.0
3.7 LIP
3.1 PANCREAS
3.0 KIDNEY
2.9 N.H.L.
18.7
28.6

F

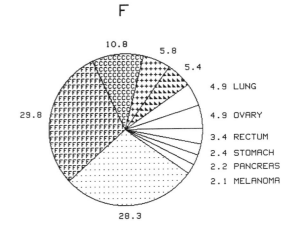

10.8   5.8
5.4
4.9 LUNG
4.9 OVARY
29.8
3.4 RECTUM
2.4 STOMACH
2.2 PANCREAS
2.1 MELANOMA
28.3

CANADA, NEWFOUNDLAND

M

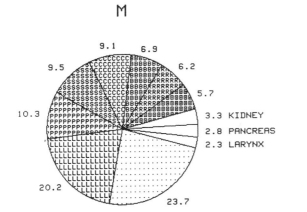

9.1   6.9
9.5   6.2
5.7
3.3 KIDNEY
2.8 PANCREAS
10.3
2.3 LARYNX
20.2
23.7

F

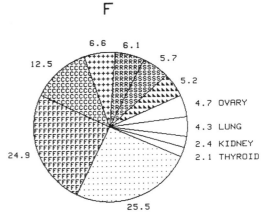

6.6   6.1
5.7
12.5
5.2
4.7 OVARY
4.3 LUNG
2.4 KIDNEY
2.1 THYROID
24.9
25.5

CANADA, NORTHWEST TERRITORIES AND YUKON

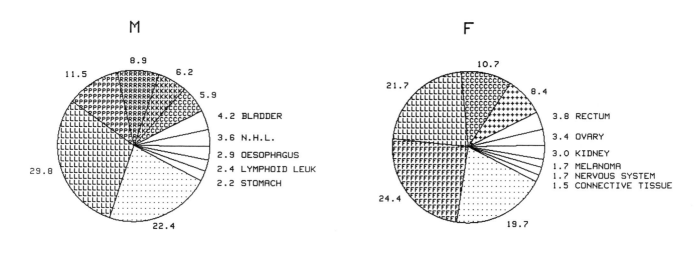

M

8.9
11.5
6.2
5.9
4.2 BLADDER
3.6 N.H.L.
2.9 OESOPHAGUS
2.4 LYMPHOID LEUK
2.2 STOMACH
29.8
22.4

F

10.7
21.7
8.4
3.8 RECTUM
3.4 OVARY
3.0 KIDNEY
1.7 MELANOMA
1.7 NERVOUS SYSTEM
1.5 CONNECTIVE TISSUE
24.4
19.7

CANADA, ONTARIO

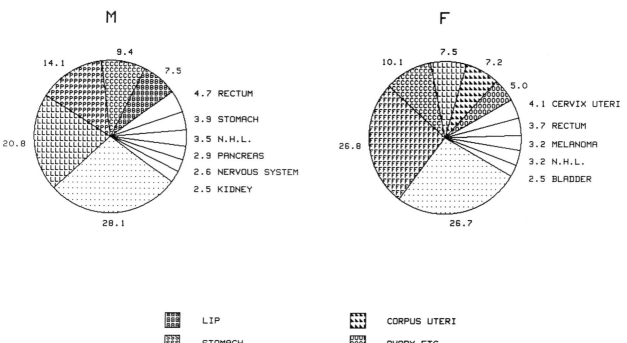

M

9.4
14.1
7.5
4.7 RECTUM
3.9 STOMACH
3.5 N.H.L.
2.9 PANCREAS
2.6 NERVOUS SYSTEM
2.5 KIDNEY
20.8
28.1

F

7.5
10.1
7.2
5.0
4.1 CERVIX UTERI
3.7 RECTUM
3.2 MELANOMA
3.2 N.H.L.
2.5 BLADDER
26.8
26.7

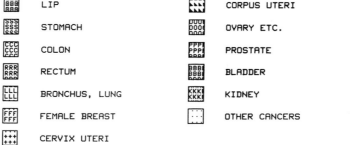

LIP
STOMACH
COLON
RECTUM
BRONCHUS, LUNG
FEMALE BREAST
CERVIX UTERI

CORPUS UTERI
OVARY ETC.
PROSTATE
BLADDER
KIDNEY
OTHER CANCERS

CANADA, QUEBEC

M

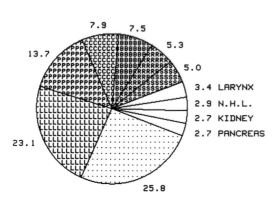

7.9   7.5
13.7   5.3
            5.0
            3.4 LARYNX
            2.9 N.H.L.
            2.7 KIDNEY
            2.7 PANCREAS
23.1
25.8

F

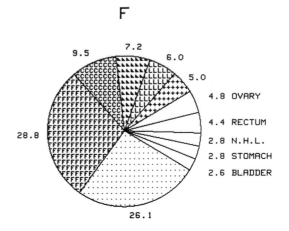

9.5   7.2   6.0
             5.0
             4.8 OVARY
             4.4 RECTUM
             2.8 N.H.L.
28.8   2.8 STOMACH
             2.6 BLADDER
26.1

CANADA, SASKATCHEWAN

M

7.2   6.3
17.3   5.9
            4.4 LIP
            4.1 STOMACH
            3.7 N.H.L.
            3.4 PANCREAS
20.4   3.1 KIDNEY
24.2

F

9.1   7.2   6.9
             5.4
             4.0 RECTUM
             3.3 N.H.L.
             3.2 CERVIX UTERI
29.8   2.7 MELANOMA
             2.6 PANCREAS
25.8

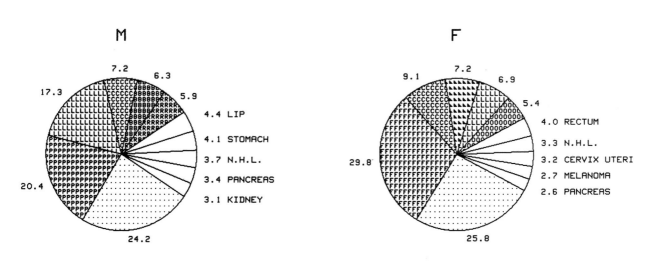

USA, CALIFORNIA, ALAMEDA COUNTY: WHITE

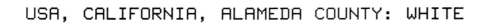

M

9.8   6.7
15.9   5.2
            3.6 N.H.L.
            3.4 STOMACH
            3.1 MELANOMA
            2.7 KIDNEY
22.0   2.7 PANCREAS
24.9

F

12.2   9.1   8.1
             4.4 OVARY
             3.9 RECTUM
             3.3 MELANOMA
             2.8 N.H.L.
28.6   2.8 CERVIX UTERI
             2.5 BLADDER
22.3

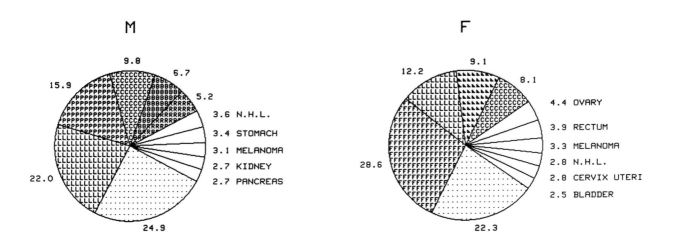

USA, CALIFORNIA, ALAMEDA COUNTY: BLACK

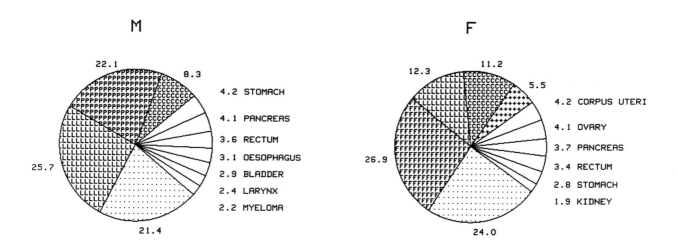

M

22.1
8.3
25.7
21.4

4.2 STOMACH
4.1 PANCREAS
3.6 RECTUM
3.1 OESOPHAGUS
2.9 BLADDER
2.4 LARYNX
2.2 MYELOMA

F

12.3
11.2
5.5
26.9
24.0

4.2 CORPUS UTERI
4.1 OVARY
3.7 PANCREAS
3.4 RECTUM
2.8 STOMACH
1.9 KIDNEY

USA, CALIFORNIA, SAN FRANCISCO BAY AREA: WHITE

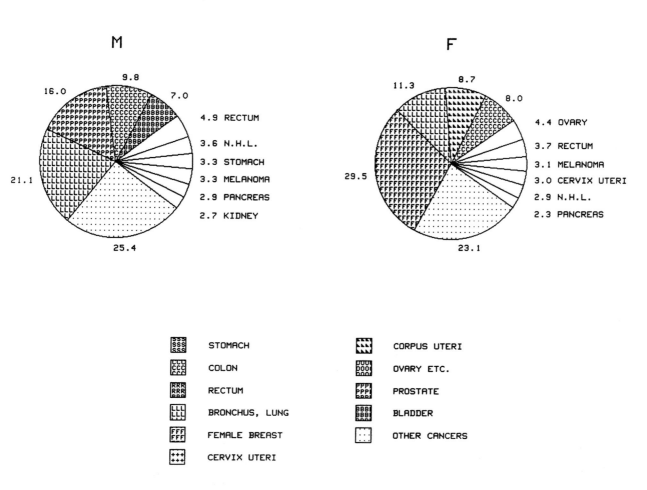

M

9.8
16.0
7.0
21.1
25.4

4.9 RECTUM
3.6 N.H.L.
3.3 STOMACH
3.3 MELANOMA
2.9 PANCREAS
2.7 KIDNEY

F

8.7
11.3
8.0
29.5
23.1

4.4 OVARY
3.7 RECTUM
3.1 MELANOMA
3.0 CERVIX UTERI
2.9 N.H.L.
2.3 PANCREAS

STOMACH   CORPUS UTERI
COLON   OVARY ETC.
RECTUM   PROSTATE
BRONCHUS, LUNG   BLADDER
FEMALE BREAST   OTHER CANCERS
CERVIX UTERI

USA, CALIFORNIA, SAN FRANCISCO BAY AREA: BLACK

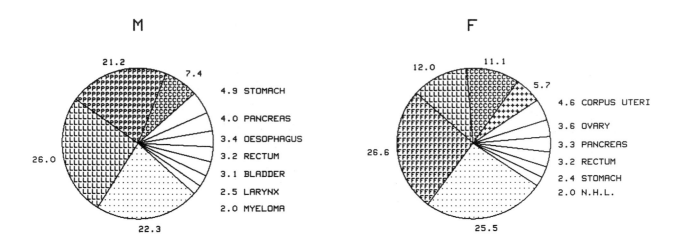

M

21.2 7.4
4.9 STOMACH
4.0 PANCREAS
3.4 OESOPHAGUS
3.2 RECTUM
3.1 BLADDER
2.5 LARYNX
2.0 MYELOMA
26.0
22.3

F

12.0 11.1 5.7
4.6 CORPUS UTERI
3.6 OVARY
3.3 PANCREAS
3.2 RECTUM
2.4 STOMACH
2.0 N.H.L.
26.6
25.5

USA, CALIFORNIA, SAN FRANCISCO BAY AREA: CHINESE

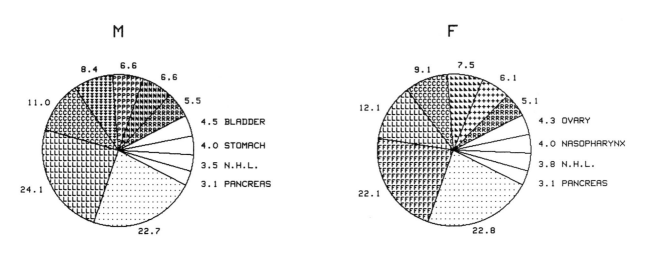

M

8.4 6.6 6.6
11.0 5.5
4.5 BLADDER
4.0 STOMACH
3.5 N.H.L.
3.1 PANCREAS
24.1
22.7

F

9.1 7.5 6.1
12.1 5.1
4.3 OVARY
4.0 NASOPHARYNX
3.8 N.H.L.
3.1 PANCREAS
22.1
22.8

USA, CALIFORNIA, SAN FRANCISCO BAY AREA: FILIPINO

M

17.9 8.4 5.6
4.4 PANCREAS
4.4 N.H.L.
3.9 RECTUM
3.1 THYROID
2.7 MYELOMA
2.5 STOMACH
19.8
27.3

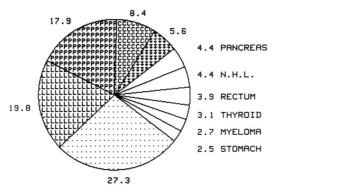

F

7.9 6.2 5.6
8.8 5.5
5.3
3.2 N.H.L.
3.0 RECTUM
1.8 PANCREAS
26.9
25.8

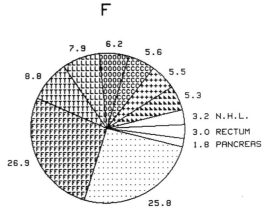

USA, CALIFORNIA, SAN FRANCISCO BAY AREA: JAPANESE

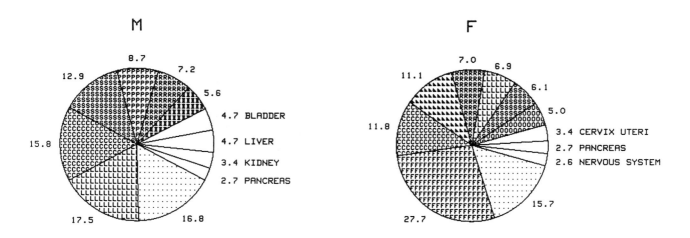

M

8.7
7.2
12.9
5.6
15.8
4.7 BLADDER
4.7 LIVER
3.4 KIDNEY
2.7 PANCREAS
17.5
16.8

F

7.0
6.9
11.1
6.1
11.8
5.0
3.4 CERVIX UTERI
2.7 PANCREAS
2.6 NERVOUS SYSTEM
27.7
15.7

USA, CALIFORNIA, LOS ANGELES COUNTY: OTHER WHITE

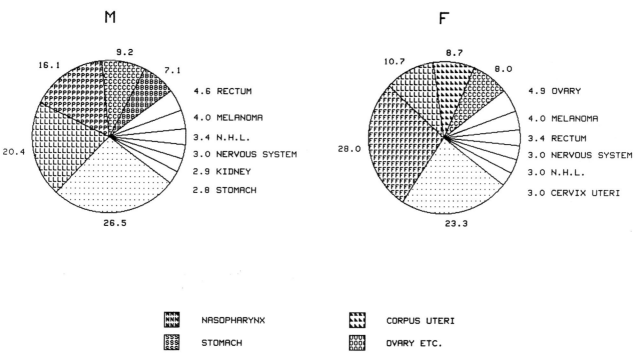

M

9.2
16.1
7.1
4.6 RECTUM
4.0 MELANOMA
3.4 N.H.L.
20.4
3.0 NERVOUS SYSTEM
2.9 KIDNEY
2.8 STOMACH
26.5

F

8.7
10.7
8.0
4.9 OVARY
4.0 MELANOMA
3.4 RECTUM
28.0
3.0 NERVOUS SYSTEM
3.0 N.H.L.
3.0 CERVIX UTERI
23.3

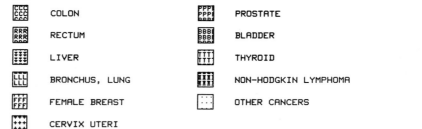

NASOPHARYNX

STOMACH

COLON

RECTUM

LIVER

BRONCHUS, LUNG

FEMALE BREAST

CERVIX UTERI

CORPUS UTERI

OVARY ETC.

PROSTATE

BLADDER

THYROID

NON-HODGKIN LYMPHOMA

OTHER CANCERS

USA, CALIFORNIA, LOS ANGELES COUNTY: LATINO

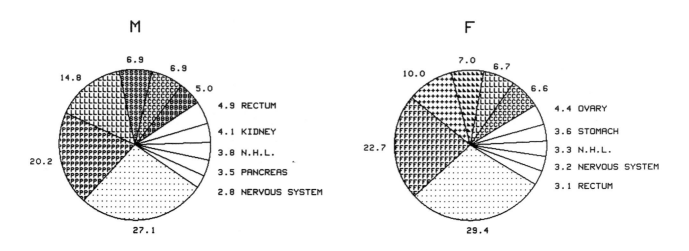

M

6.9
6.9
14.8
5.0
4.9 RECTUM
4.1 KIDNEY
3.8 N.H.L.
20.2
3.5 PANCREAS
2.8 NERVOUS SYSTEM
27.1

F

7.0
6.7
10.0
6.6
4.4 OVARY
3.6 STOMACH
3.3 N.H.L.
3.2 NERVOUS SYSTEM
22.7
3.1 RECTUM
29.4

USA, CALIFORNIA, LOS ANGELES COUNTY: BLACK

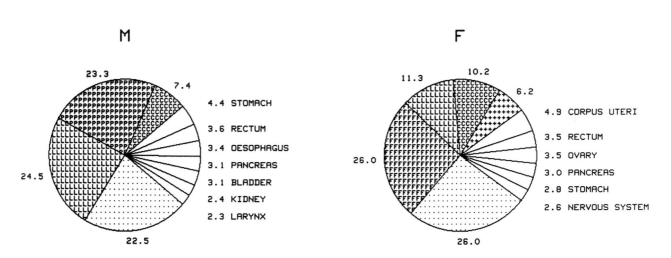

M

23.3
7.4
4.4 STOMACH
3.6 RECTUM
3.4 OESOPHAGUS
3.1 PANCREAS
3.1 BLADDER
24.5
2.4 KIDNEY
2.3 LARYNX
22.5

F

11.3
10.2
6.2
4.9 CORPUS UTERI
3.5 RECTUM
3.5 OVARY
3.0 PANCREAS
26.0
2.8 STOMACH
2.6 NERVOUS SYSTEM
26.0

USA, CALIFORNIA, LOS ANGELES COUNTY: JAPANESE

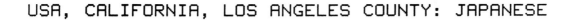

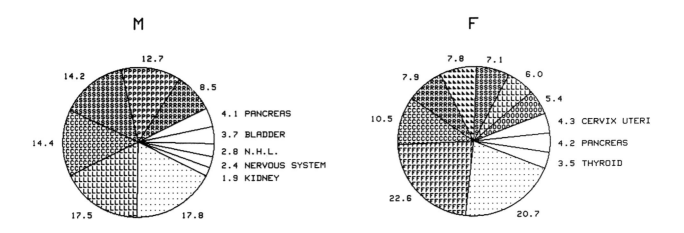

M

12.7
14.2
8.5
4.1 PANCREAS
3.7 BLADDER
2.8 N.H.L.
14.4
2.4 NERVOUS SYSTEM
1.9 KIDNEY
17.5
17.8

F

7.8
7.1
7.9
6.0
5.4
10.5
4.3 CERVIX UTERI
4.2 PANCREAS
3.5 THYROID
22.6
20.7

USA, CALIFORNIA, LOS ANGELES COUNTY: CHINESE

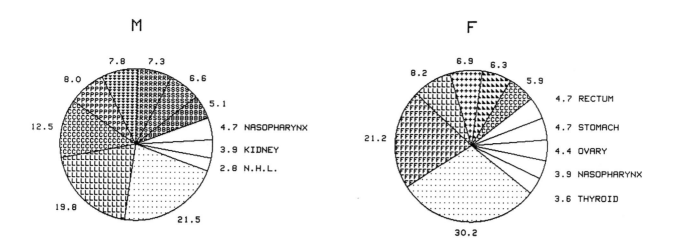

M

7.8 7.3
8.0 6.6
5.1
4.7 NASOPHARYNX
12.5
3.9 KIDNEY
2.8 N.H.L.
19.8
21.5

F

6.9 6.3
8.2 5.9
4.7 RECTUM
4.7 STOMACH
21.2
4.4 OVARY
3.9 NASOPHARYNX
3.6 THYROID
30.2

USA, CALIFORNIA, LOS ANGELES COUNTY: FILIPINO

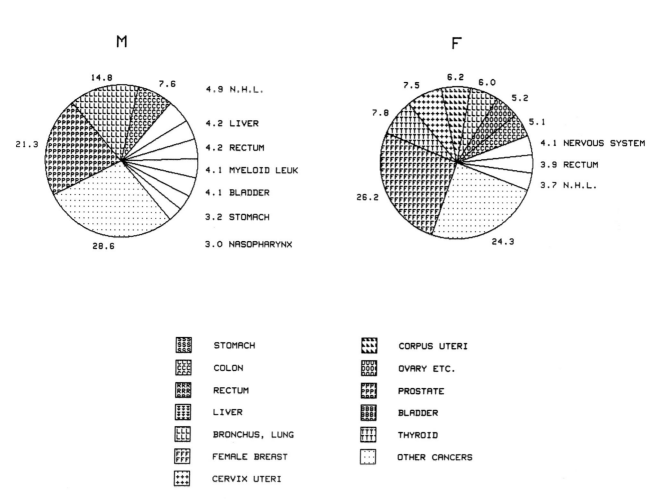

M

14.8 7.6
4.9 N.H.L.
4.2 LIVER
21.3
4.2 RECTUM
4.1 MYELOID LEUK
4.1 BLADDER
3.2 STOMACH
28.6
3.0 NASOPHARYNX

F

7.5 6.2 6.0
5.2
7.8
5.1
4.1 NERVOUS SYSTEM
3.9 RECTUM
26.2
3.7 N.H.L.
24.3

STOMACH		CORPUS UTERI
COLON		OVARY ETC.
RECTUM		PROSTATE
LIVER		BLADDER
BRONCHUS, LUNG		THYROID
FEMALE BREAST		OTHER CANCERS
CERVIX UTERI		

USA, CALIFORNIA, LOS ANGELES COUNTY: KOREAN

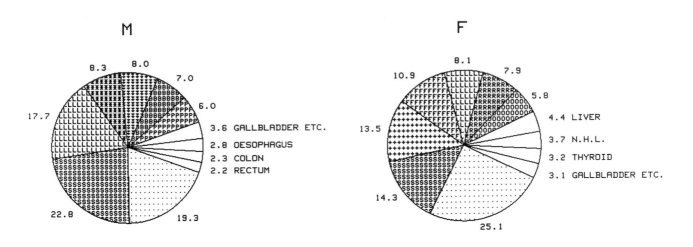

M

F

8.3 8.0 7.0
6.0
17.7
3.6 GALLBLADDER ETC.
2.8 OESOPHAGUS
2.3 COLON
2.2 RECTUM
22.8 19.3

8.1 7.9
10.9 5.8
13.5
4.4 LIVER
3.7 N.H.L.
3.2 THYROID
3.1 GALLBLADDER ETC.
14.3 25.1

USA, CONNECTICUT: WHITE

M

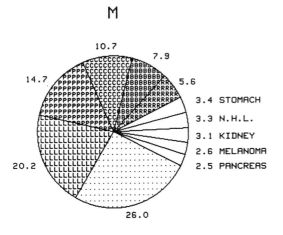

10.7 7.9
14.7 5.6
3.4 STOMACH
3.3 N.H.L.
3.1 KIDNEY
2.6 MELANOMA
20.2 2.5 PANCREAS
26.0

F

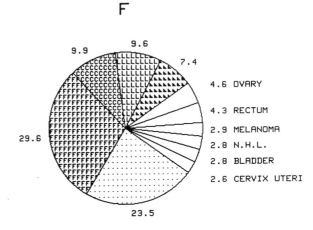

9.9 9.6 7.4
4.6 OVARY
4.3 RECTUM
2.9 MELANOMA
29.6 2.8 N.H.L.
2.8 BLADDER
2.6 CERVIX UTERI
23.5

USA, CONNECTICUT: BLACK

M

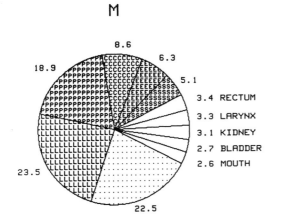

8.6 6.3
18.9 5.1
3.4 RECTUM
3.3 LARYNX
3.1 KIDNEY
2.7 BLADDER
23.5 2.6 MOUTH
22.5

F

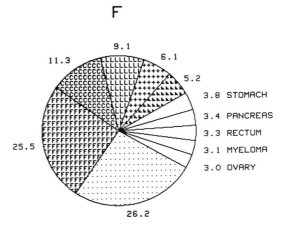

9.1 6.1
11.3 5.2
3.8 STOMACH
3.4 PANCREAS
3.3 RECTUM
25.5 3.1 MYELOMA
3.0 OVARY
26.2

USA, GEORGIA, ATLANTA: WHITE

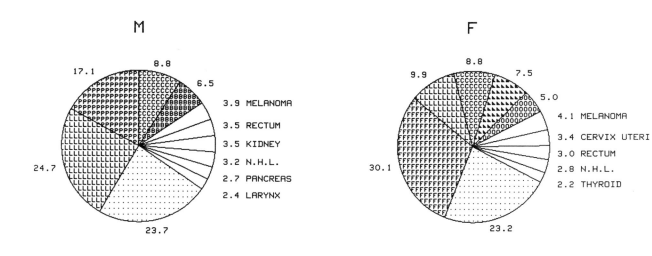

M

8.8
17.1
6.5

3.9 MELANOMA
3.5 RECTUM
3.5 KIDNEY
3.2 N.H.L.
2.7 PANCREAS
2.4 LARYNX

24.7

23.7

F

8.8
9.9
7.5
5.0

4.1 MELANOMA
3.4 CERVIX UTERI
3.0 RECTUM
2.8 N.H.L.
2.2 THYROID

30.1

23.2

USA, GEORGIA, ATLANTA: BLACK

M

24.6
6.5

4.6 OESOPHAGUS
4.3 STOMACH
3.2 PANCREAS
3.1 LARYNX
2.9 BLADDER
2.2 RECTUM
2.1 MYELOMA

25.5

21.0

F

8.9
10.6
7.1
5.4

4.1 PANCREAS
3.9 OVARY
3.3 RECTUM
2.6 STOMACH
2.4 MYELOMA

26.5

25.2

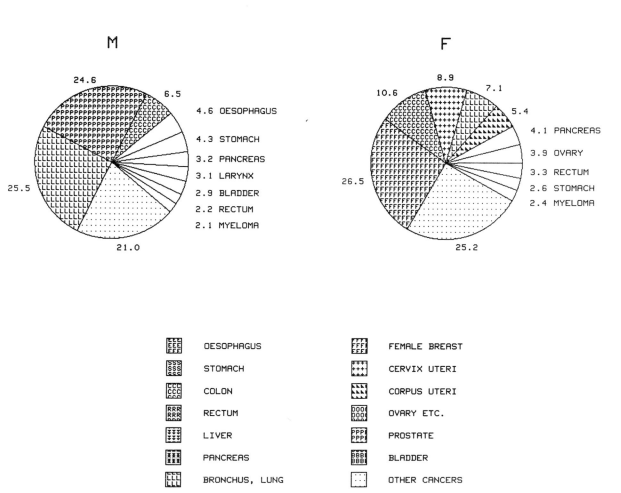

OESOPHAGUS	FEMALE BREAST
STOMACH	CERVIX UTERI
COLON	CORPUS UTERI
RECTUM	OVARY ETC.
LIVER	PROSTATE
PANCREAS	BLADDER
BRONCHUS, LUNG	OTHER CANCERS

USA, IOWA

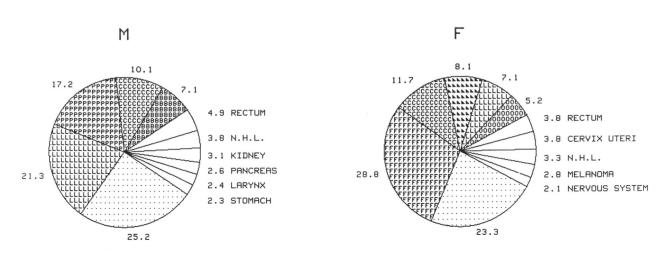

M

10.1
17.2
7.1

4.9 RECTUM
3.8 N.H.L.
3.1 KIDNEY
2.6 PANCREAS
2.4 LARYNX
2.3 STOMACH

21.3

25.2

F

8.1
11.7
7.1
5.2

3.8 RECTUM
3.8 CERVIX UTERI
3.3 N.H.L.
2.8 MELANOMA
2.1 NERVOUS SYSTEM

28.8

23.3

USA, LOUISIANA, NEW ORLEANS: WHITE

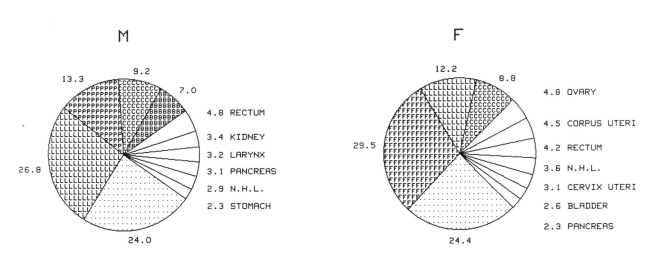

M

9.2
13.3
7.0

4.8 RECTUM
3.4 KIDNEY
3.2 LARYNX
3.1 PANCREAS
2.9 N.H.L.
2.3 STOMACH

26.8

24.0

F

12.2
8.8

4.8 OVARY
4.5 CORPUS UTERI
4.2 RECTUM
3.6 N.H.L.
3.1 CERVIX UTERI
2.6 BLADDER
2.3 PANCREAS

29.5

24.4

USA, LOUISIANA, NEW ORLEANS: BLACK

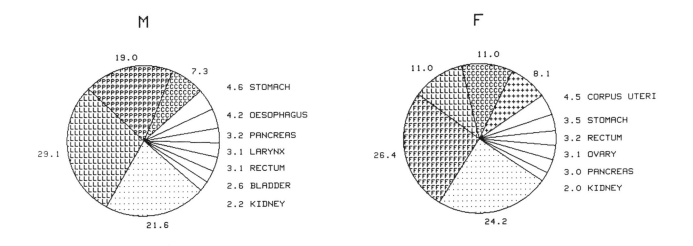

M

19.0
7.3

4.6 STOMACH
4.2 OESOPHAGUS
3.2 PANCREAS
3.1 LARYNX
3.1 RECTUM
2.6 BLADDER
2.2 KIDNEY

29.1

21.6

F

11.0
11.0
8.1

4.5 CORPUS UTERI
3.5 STOMACH
3.2 RECTUM
3.1 OVARY
3.0 PANCREAS
2.0 KIDNEY

26.4

24.2

USA, MICHIGAN, DETROIT: WHITE

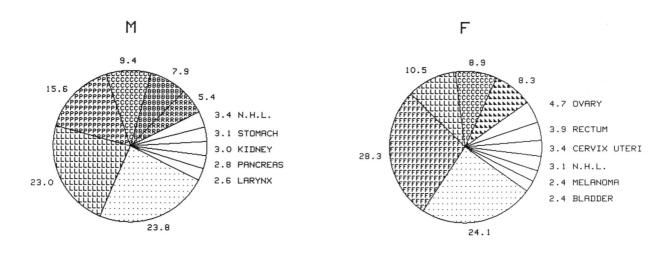

M

9.4
7.9
15.6
5.4
3.4 N.H.L.
3.1 STOMACH
3.0 KIDNEY
2.8 PANCREAS
2.6 LARYNX
23.0
23.8

F

8.9
10.5
8.3
4.7 OVARY
3.9 RECTUM
3.4 CERVIX UTERI
3.1 N.H.L.
2.4 MELANOMA
2.4 BLADDER
28.3
24.1

USA, MICHIGAN, DETROIT: BLACK

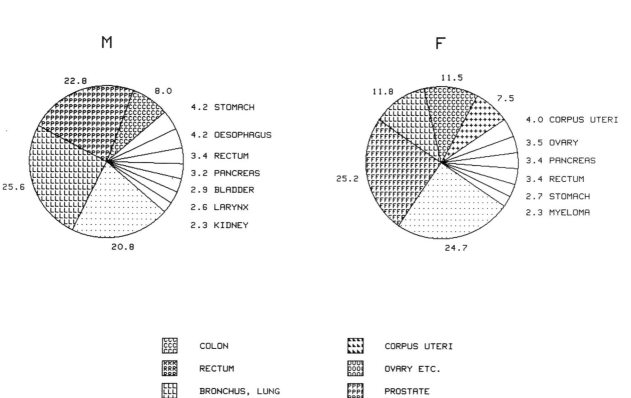

M

22.8
8.0
4.2 STOMACH
4.2 OESOPHAGUS
3.4 RECTUM
3.2 PANCREAS
2.9 BLADDER
2.6 LARYNX
2.3 KIDNEY
25.6
20.8

F

11.5
11.8
7.5
4.0 CORPUS UTERI
3.5 OVARY
3.4 PANCREAS
3.4 RECTUM
2.7 STOMACH
2.3 MYELOMA
25.2
24.7

COLON		CORPUS UTERI
RECTUM		OVARY ETC.
BRONCHUS, LUNG		PROSTATE
FEMALE BREAST		BLADDER
CERVIX UTERI		OTHER CANCERS

USA, NEW MEXICO: HISPANIC

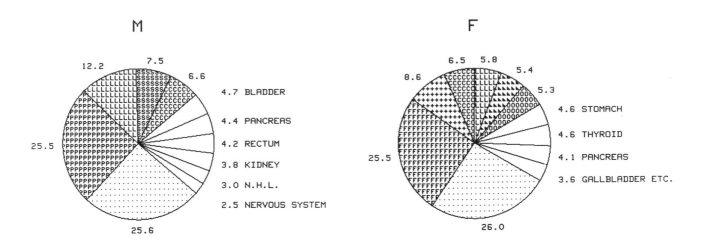

M

12.2   7.5

6.6

25.5

25.6

4.7 BLADDER
4.4 PANCREAS
4.2 RECTUM
3.8 KIDNEY
3.0 N.H.L.
2.5 NERVOUS SYSTEM

F

6.5   5.8

8.6

5.4

5.3

25.5

26.0

4.6 STOMACH
4.6 THYROID
4.1 PANCREAS
3.6 GALLBLADDER ETC.

USA, NEW MEXICO: OTHER WHITE (ANGLO)

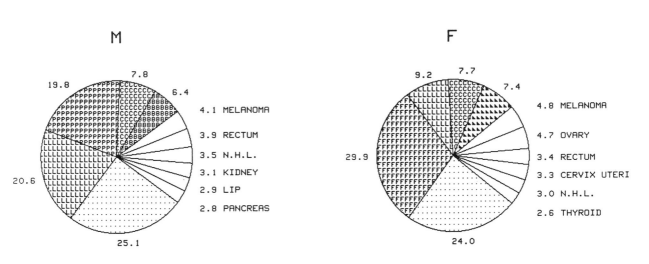

M

7.8

19.8

6.4

20.6

25.1

4.1 MELANOMA
3.9 RECTUM
3.5 N.H.L.
3.1 KIDNEY
2.9 LIP
2.8 PANCREAS

F

9.2   7.7

7.4

29.9

24.0

4.8 MELANOMA
4.7 OVARY
3.4 RECTUM
3.3 CERVIX UTERI
3.0 N.H.L.
2.6 THYROID

USA, NEW MEXICO: AMERICAN INDIAN

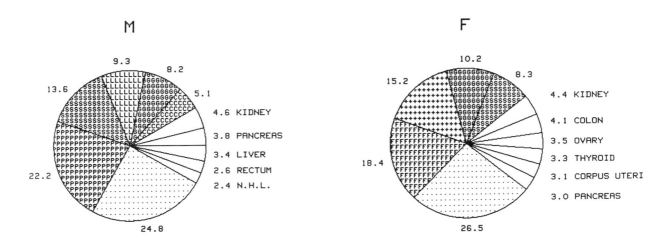

M

9.3   8.2

13.6

5.1

22.2

24.8

4.6 KIDNEY
3.8 PANCREAS
3.4 LIVER
2.6 RECTUM
2.4 N.H.L.

F

10.2

15.2

8.3

18.4

26.5

4.4 KIDNEY
4.1 COLON
3.5 OVARY
3.3 THYROID
3.1 CORPUS UTERI
3.0 PANCREAS

USA, NEW YORK CITY

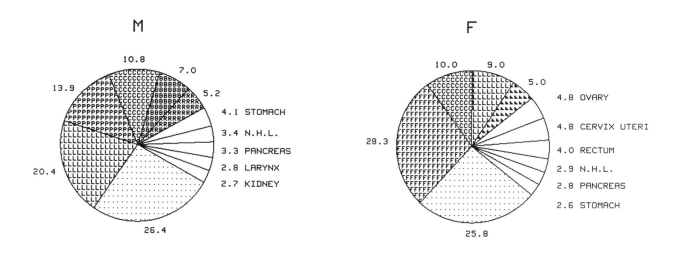

M

10.8
7.0
13.9
5.2
4.1 STOMACH
3.4 N.H.L.
3.3 PANCREAS
2.8 LARYNX
2.7 KIDNEY
20.4
26.4

F

10.0 9.0
5.0
4.8 OVARY
4.8 CERVIX UTERI
4.0 RECTUM
2.9 N.H.L.
2.8 PANCREAS
2.6 STOMACH
28.3
25.8

USA, NEW YORK STATE (LESS NEW YORK CITY)

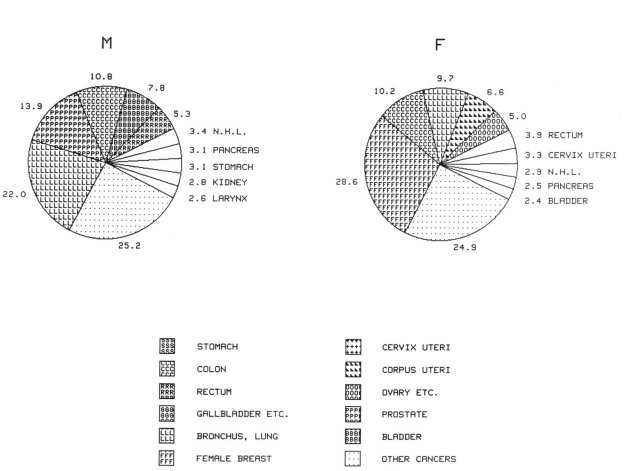

M

10.8
7.8
13.9
5.3
3.4 N.H.L.
3.1 PANCREAS
3.1 STOMACH
2.8 KIDNEY
2.6 LARYNX
22.0
25.2

F

9.7
10.2 6.6
5.0
3.9 RECTUM
3.3 CERVIX UTERI
2.9 N.H.L.
2.5 PANCREAS
2.4 BLADDER
28.6
24.9

STOMACH		CERVIX UTERI	
COLON		CORPUS UTERI	
RECTUM		OVARY ETC.	
GALLBLADDER ETC.		PROSTATE	
BRONCHUS, LUNG		BLADDER	
FEMALE BREAST		OTHER CANCERS	

75

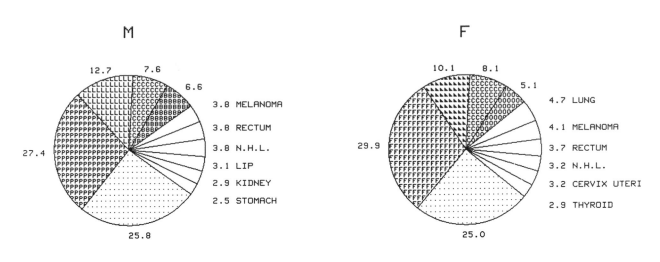

M

F

12.7 7.6
6.6
3.8 MELANOMA
3.8 RECTUM
3.8 N.H.L.
27.4   3.1 LIP
2.9 KIDNEY
2.5 STOMACH
25.8

10.1 8.1
5.1
4.7 LUNG
4.1 MELANOMA
3.7 RECTUM
29.9   3.2 N.H.L.
3.2 CERVIX UTERI
2.9 THYROID
25.0

USA, WASHINGTON, SEATTLE

M

F

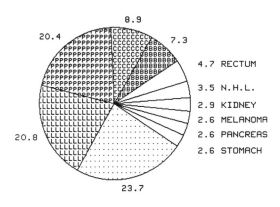

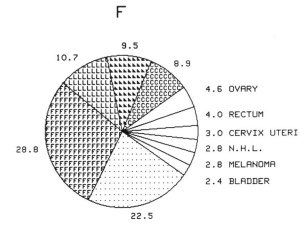

8.9
20.4   7.3
4.7 RECTUM
3.5 N.H.L.
2.9 KIDNEY
2.6 MELANOMA
20.8   2.6 PANCREAS
2.6 STOMACH
23.7

9.5
10.7   8.9
4.6 OVARY
4.0 RECTUM
3.0 CERVIX UTERI
28.8   2.8 N.H.L.
2.8 MELANOMA
2.4 BLADDER
22.5

CHINA, SHANGHAI

M

F

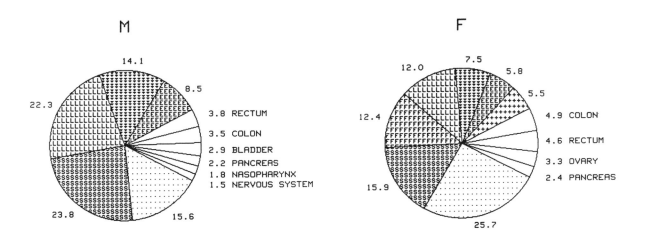

14.1
22.3   8.5
3.8 RECTUM
3.5 COLON
2.9 BLADDER
2.2 PANCREAS
1.8 NASOPHARYNX
1.5 NERVOUS SYSTEM
23.8   15.6

7.5
12.0   5.8
5.5
12.4   4.9 COLON
4.6 RECTUM
3.3 OVARY
2.4 PANCREAS
15.9
25.7

CHINA, TIANJIN

M

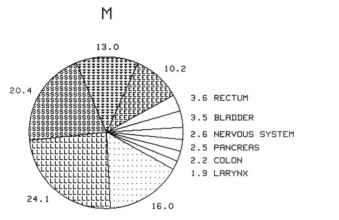

13.0
10.2
20.4
3.6 RECTUM
3.5 BLADDER
2.6 NERVOUS SYSTEM
2.5 PANCREAS
2.2 COLON
1.9 LARYNX
24.1
16.0

F

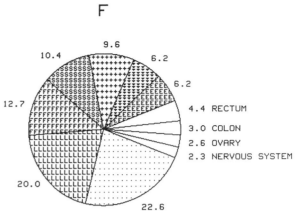

9.6
10.4
6.2
6.2
12.7
4.4 RECTUM
3.0 COLON
2.6 OVARY
2.3 NERVOUS SYSTEM
20.0
22.6

HONG KONG

M

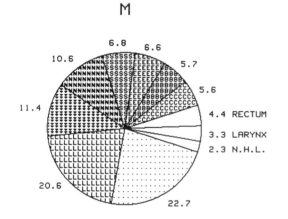

6.8
6.6
10.6
5.7
5.6
11.4
4.4 RECTUM
3.3 LARYNX
2.3 N.H.L.
20.6
22.7

F

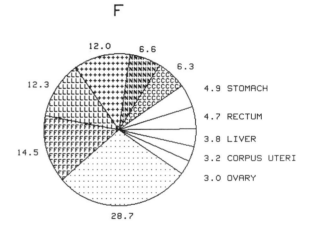

12.0
6.6
12.3
6.3
4.9 STOMACH
4.7 RECTUM
3.8 LIVER
14.5
3.2 CORPUS UTERI
3.0 OVARY
28.7

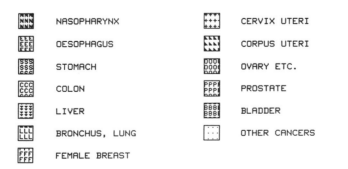

NASOPHARYNX	CERVIX UTERI
OESOPHAGUS	CORPUS UTERI
STOMACH	OVARY ETC.
COLON	PROSTATE
LIVER	BLADDER
BRONCHUS, LUNG	OTHER CANCERS
FEMALE BREAST	

INDIA, BANGALORE

M

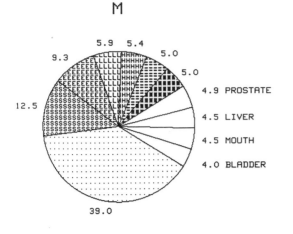

5.9 5.4
9.3   5.0
5.0
12.5
4.9 PROSTATE
4.5 LIVER
4.5 MOUTH
4.0 BLADDER
39.0

F

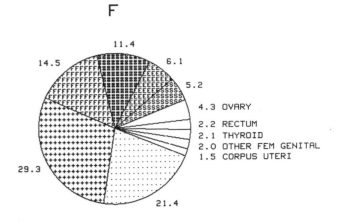

11.4
14.5   6.1
5.2
4.3 OVARY
2.2 RECTUM
2.1 THYROID
2.0 OTHER FEM GENITAL
1.5 CORPUS UTERI
29.3
21.4

INDIA, BOMBAY

M

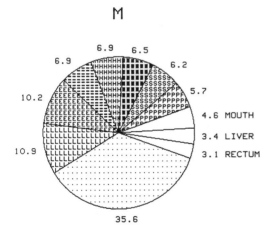

6.9 6.5
6.9   6.2
10.2   5.7
4.6 MOUTH
3.4 LIVER
3.1 RECTUM
10.9
35.6

F

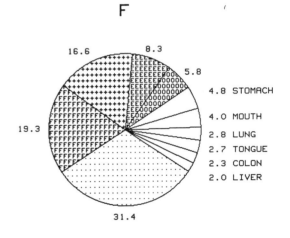

16.6   8.3
5.8
4.8 STOMACH
4.0 MOUTH
2.8 LUNG
2.7 TONGUE
2.3 COLON
2.0 LIVER
19.3
31.4

INDIA, MADRAS

M

8.5   6.3
8.8   5.8
4.8 TONGUE
4.6 HYPOPHARYNX
3.7 PENIS ETC.
3.4 PROSTATE
3.3 RECTUM
15.0
35.8

F

17.4   8.3
5.6
3.6 OVARY
3.2 OESOPHAGUS
1.7 TONGUE
1.6 OTHER FEM GENITAL
1.6 CORPUS UTERI
1.5 THYROID
38.5
17.0

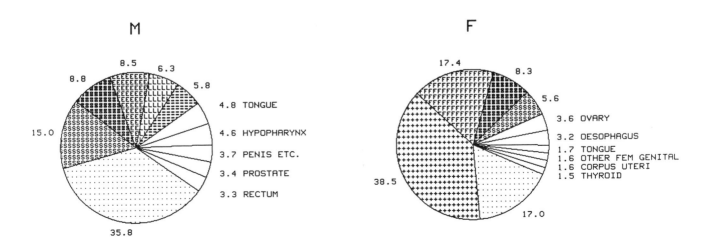

INDIA, NAGPUR

M

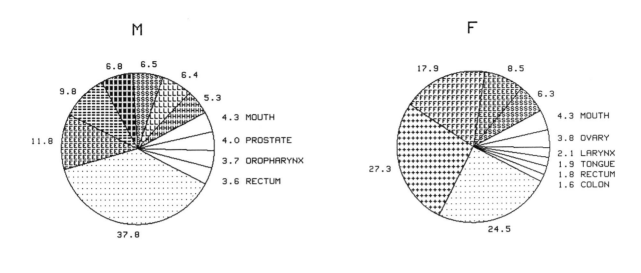

6.8 6.5
6.4
9.8
5.3
4.3 MOUTH
4.0 PROSTATE
11.8
3.7 OROPHARYNX
3.6 RECTUM
37.8

F

17.9 8.5
6.3
4.3 MOUTH
3.8 OVARY
2.1 LARYNX
27.3
1.9 TONGUE
1.8 RECTUM
1.6 COLON
24.5

INDIA, POONA

M

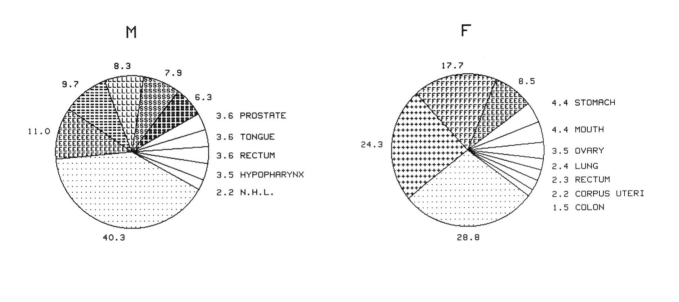

8.3 7.9
9.7
6.3
3.6 PROSTATE
3.6 TONGUE
11.0
3.6 RECTUM
3.5 HYPOPHARYNX
2.2 N.H.L.
40.3

F

17.7 8.5
4.4 STOMACH
4.4 MOUTH
3.5 OVARY
24.3
2.4 LUNG
2.3 RECTUM
2.2 CORPUS UTERI
1.5 COLON
28.8

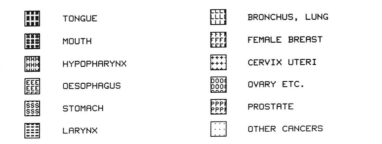

TONGUE

MOUTH

HYPOPHARYNX

OESOPHAGUS

STOMACH

LARYNX

BRONCHUS, LUNG

FEMALE BREAST

CERVIX UTERI

OVARY ETC.

PROSTATE

OTHER CANCERS

ISRAEL: ALL JEWS

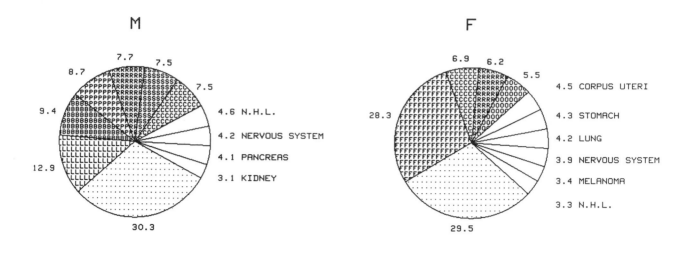

ISRAEL: JEWS BORN IN ISRAEL

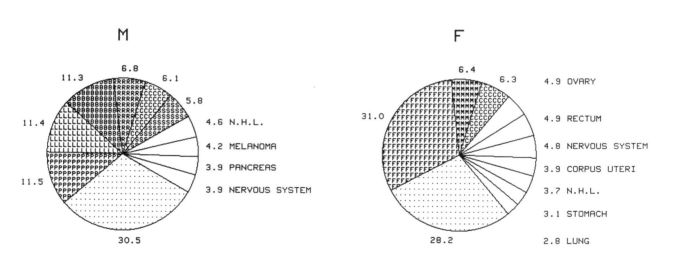

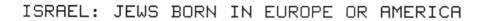

ISRAEL: JEWS BORN IN EUROPE OR AMERICA

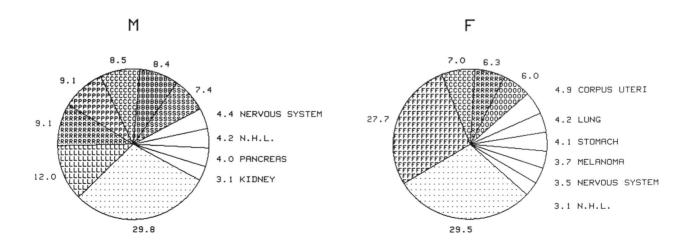

ISRAEL: JEWS BORN IN AFRICA OR ASIA

M

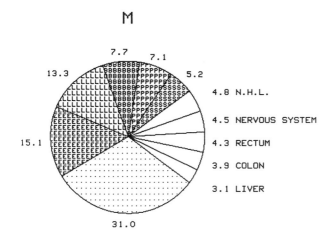

7.7 7.1
13.3 5.2
4.8 N.H.L.
4.5 NERVOUS SYSTEM
15.1 4.3 RECTUM
3.9 COLON
3.1 LIVER
31.0

F

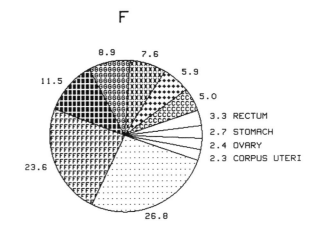

8.9 7.6 5.9
11.5 5.0
3.3 RECTUM
2.7 STOMACH
2.4 OVARY
23.6 2.3 CORPUS UTERI
26.8

ISRAEL: NON-JEWS

M

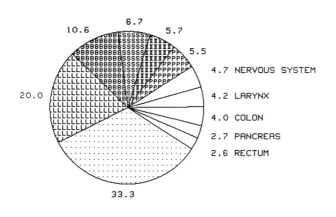

6.7
10.6 5.7 5.5
4.7 NERVOUS SYSTEM
4.2 LARYNX
20.0 4.0 COLON
2.7 PANCREAS
2.6 RECTUM
33.3

F

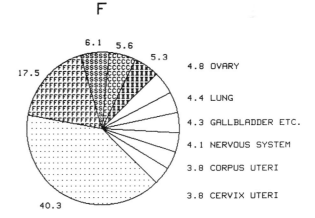

6.1 5.6
5.3
17.5 4.8 OVARY
4.4 LUNG
4.3 GALLBLADDER ETC.
4.1 NERVOUS SYSTEM
3.8 CORPUS UTERI
3.8 CERVIX UTERI
40.3

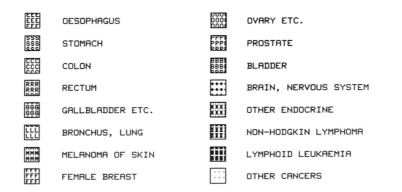

OESOPHAGUS		OVARY ETC.
STOMACH		PROSTATE
COLON		BLADDER
RECTUM		BRAIN, NERVOUS SYSTEM
GALLBLADDER ETC.		OTHER ENDOCRINE
BRONCHUS, LUNG		NON-HODGKIN LYMPHOMA
MELANOMA OF SKIN		LYMPHOID LEUKAEMIA
FEMALE BREAST		OTHER CANCERS

JAPAN, HIROSHIMA CITY

M

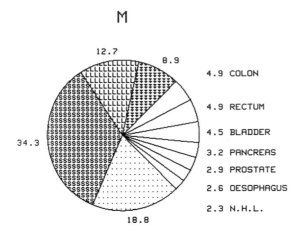

12.7   8.9
34.3
18.8

4.9 COLON
4.9 RECTUM
4.5 BLADDER
3.2 PANCREAS
2.9 PROSTATE
2.6 OESOPHAGUS
2.3 N.H.L.

F

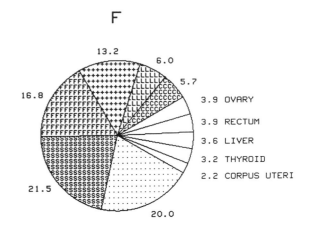

13.2   6.0
16.8   5.7
21.5
20.0

3.9 OVARY
3.9 RECTUM
3.6 LIVER
3.2 THYROID
2.2 CORPUS UTERI

JAPAN, MIYAGI PREFECTURE

M

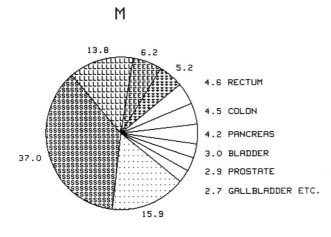

13.8   6.2
5.2
37.0
15.9

4.6 RECTUM
4.5 COLON
4.2 PANCREAS
3.0 BLADDER
2.9 PROSTATE
2.7 GALLBLADDER ETC.

F

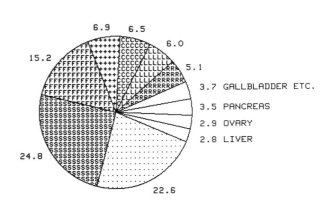

6.9   6.5
15.2   6.0
5.1
24.8
22.6

3.7 GALLBLADDER ETC.
3.5 PANCREAS
2.9 OVARY
2.8 LIVER

JAPAN, NAGASAKI CITY

M

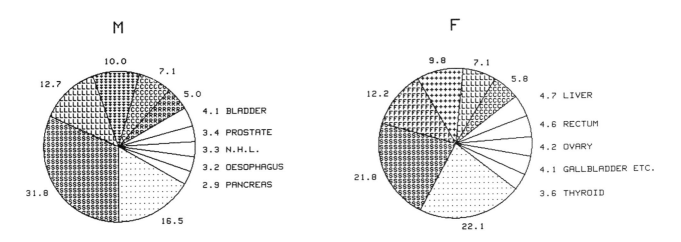

10.0   7.1
12.7   5.0
31.8
16.5

4.1 BLADDER
3.4 PROSTATE
3.3 N.H.L.
3.2 OESOPHAGUS
2.9 PANCREAS

F

9.8   7.1
12.2   5.8
21.8
22.1

4.7 LIVER
4.6 RECTUM
4.2 OVARY
4.1 GALLBLADDER ETC.
3.6 THYROID

82

JAPAN, OSAKA PREFECTURE

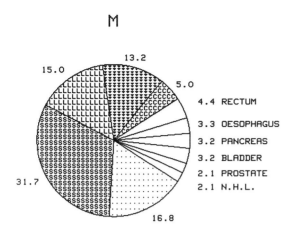

M

15.0   13.2
                5.0
         4.4 RECTUM
         3.3 OESOPHAGUS
         3.2 PANCREAS
         3.2 BLADDER
         2.1 PROSTATE
         2.1 N.H.L.
31.7
         16.8

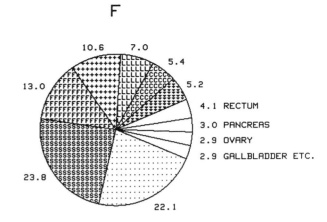

F

10.6   7.0
              5.4
13.0   5.2
         4.1 RECTUM
         3.0 PANCREAS
         2.9 OVARY
         2.9 GALLBLADDER ETC.
23.8
         22.1

KUWAIT: KUWAITIS

M

8.3   6.2
         6.1
            5.1
         4.7 LARYNX
19.2
         4.1 RECTUM
         4.0 N.H.L.
         2.9 NASOPHARYNX
         2.8 OESOPHAGUS
         36.6

F

8.8   8.8
            5.4
22.0
         4.6 OVARY
         2.8 OESOPHAGUS
         2.8 HYPOPHARYNX
         2.5 N.H.L.
         2.5 CORPUS UTERI
         2.5 MYELOID LEUK
         37.3

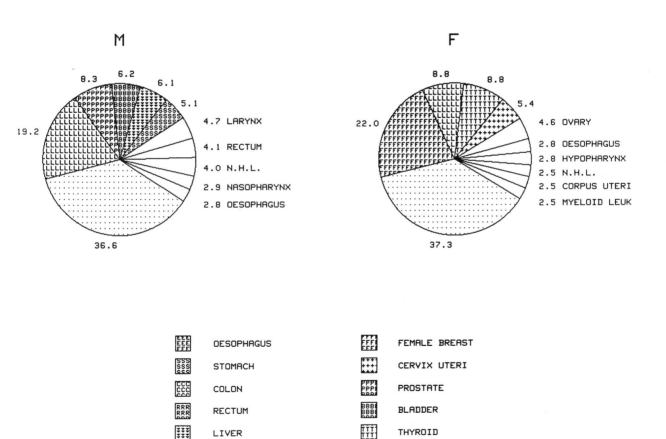

OESOPHAGUS		FEMALE BREAST
STOMACH		CERVIX UTERI
COLON		PROSTATE
RECTUM		BLADDER
LIVER		THYROID
BRONCHUS, LUNG		OTHER CANCERS

KUWAIT: NON-KUWAITIS

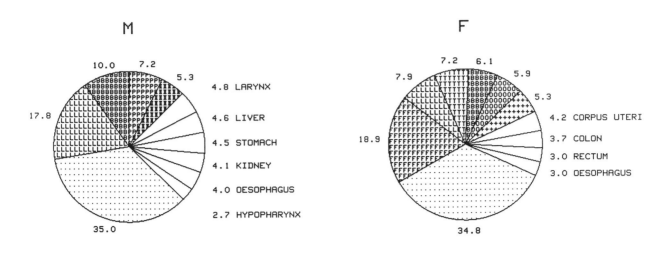

M	F
10.0 7.2	7.2 6.1
5.3	7.9 5.9
17.8	5.3
4.8 LARYNX	18.9
4.6 LIVER	4.2 CORPUS UTERI
4.5 STOMACH	3.7 COLON
4.1 KIDNEY	3.0 RECTUM
4.0 OESOPHAGUS	3.0 OESOPHAGUS
2.7 HYPOPHARYNX	
35.0	34.8

PHILIPPINES, RIZAL PROVINCE

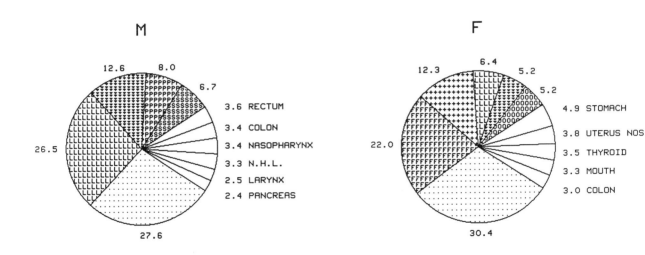

M	F
12.6 8.0	12.3 6.4 5.2
6.7	5.2
26.5	22.0
3.6 RECTUM	4.9 STOMACH
3.4 COLON	3.8 UTERUS NOS
3.4 NASOPHARYNX	3.5 THYROID
3.3 N.H.L.	3.3 MOUTH
2.5 LARYNX	3.0 COLON
2.4 PANCREAS	
27.6	30.4

SINGAPORE: CHINESE

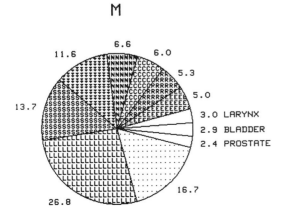
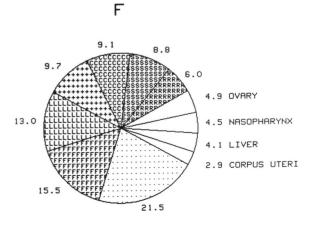

M	F
6.6 6.0	9.1 8.8
11.6 5.3	9.7 6.0
5.0	13.0
13.7	4.9 OVARY
3.0 LARYNX	4.5 NASOPHARYNX
2.9 BLADDER	4.1 LIVER
2.4 PROSTATE	2.9 CORPUS UTERI
16.7	15.5
26.8	21.5

SINGAPORE: MALAY

M

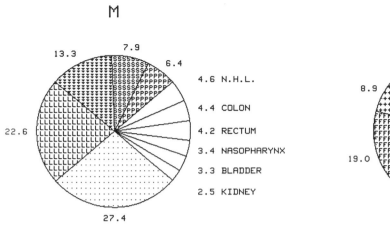

13.3 7.9
6.4
4.6 N.H.L.
4.4 COLON
4.2 RECTUM
3.4 NASOPHARYNX
3.3 BLADDER
2.5 KIDNEY
22.6
27.4

F

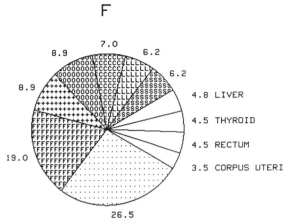

8.9 7.0 6.2
6.2
4.8 LIVER
4.5 THYROID
4.5 RECTUM
3.5 CORPUS UTERI
8.9
19.0
26.5

SINGAPORE: INDIAN

M

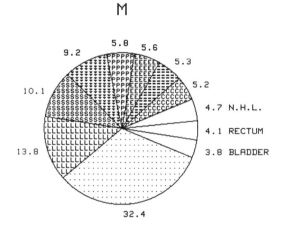

5.8 5.6
9.2
5.3
5.2
10.1
4.7 N.H.L.
4.1 RECTUM
3.8 BLADDER
13.8
32.4

F

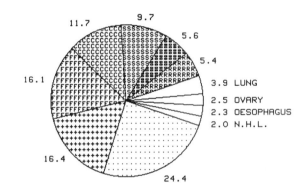

11.7 9.7
5.6
5.4
16.1
3.9 LUNG
2.5 OVARY
2.3 OESOPHAGUS
2.0 N.H.L.
16.4
24.4

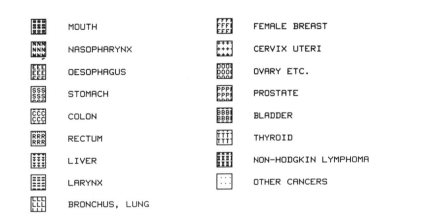

MOUTH	FEMALE BREAST
NASOPHARYNX	CERVIX UTERI
OESOPHAGUS	OVARY ETC.
STOMACH	PROSTATE
COLON	BLADDER
RECTUM	THYROID
LIVER	NON-HODGKIN LYMPHOMA
LARYNX	OTHER CANCERS
BRONCHUS, LUNG	

85

CZECHOSLOVAKIA, SLOVAKIA

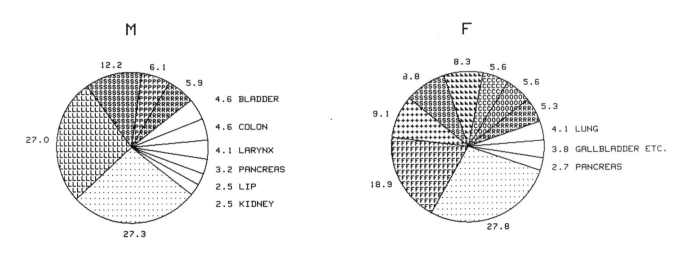

M

12.2 6.1
5.9
4.6 BLADDER
4.6 COLON
4.1 LARYNX
3.2 PANCREAS
2.5 LIP
2.5 KIDNEY
27.0
27.3

F

8.3 5.6
8.8
5.6
9.1
5.3
4.1 LUNG
3.8 GALLBLADDER ETC.
2.7 PANCREAS
18.9
27.8

DENMARK

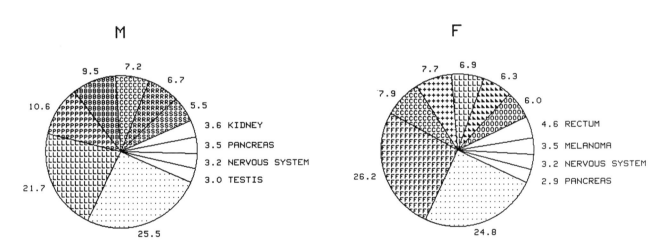

M

9.5 7.2
6.7
10.6
5.5
3.6 KIDNEY
3.5 PANCREAS
3.2 NERVOUS SYSTEM
3.0 TESTIS
21.7
25.5

F

7.7 6.9
6.3
7.9
6.0
4.6 RECTUM
3.5 MELANOMA
3.2 NERVOUS SYSTEM
2.9 PANCREAS
26.2
24.8

FEDERAL REPUBLIC OF GERMANY, HAMBURG

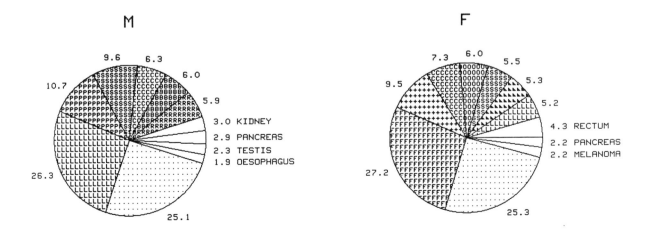

M

9.6 6.3
6.0
10.7
5.9
3.0 KIDNEY
2.9 PANCREAS
2.3 TESTIS
1.9 OESOPHAGUS
26.3
25.1

F

7.3 6.0
5.5
9.5
5.3
5.2
4.3 RECTUM
2.2 PANCREAS
2.2 MELANOMA
27.2
25.3

FEDERAL REPUBLIC OF GERMANY, SAARLAND

M

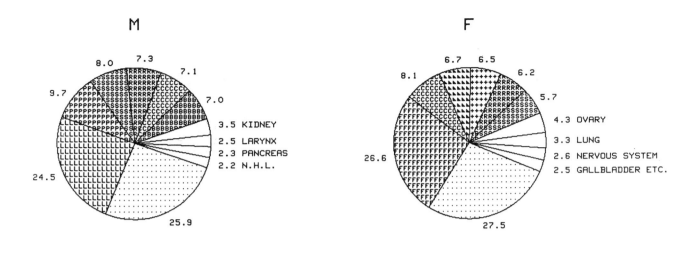

8.0 7.3 7.1 9.7 7.0
3.5 KIDNEY
2.5 LARYNX
2.3 PANCREAS
2.2 N.H.L.
24.5
25.9

F

6.7 6.5 6.2 8.1 5.7
4.3 OVARY
3.3 LUNG
2.6 NERVOUS SYSTEM
2.5 GALLBLADDER ETC.
26.6
27.5

FINLAND

M

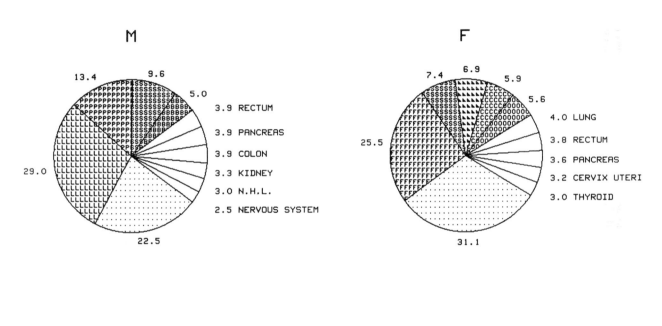

13.4 9.6 5.0
3.9 RECTUM
3.9 PANCREAS
3.9 COLON
3.3 KIDNEY
3.0 N.H.L.
2.5 NERVOUS SYSTEM
29.0
22.5

F

7.4 6.9 5.9 5.6
4.0 LUNG
3.8 RECTUM
3.6 PANCREAS
3.2 CERVIX UTERI
3.0 THYROID
25.5
31.1

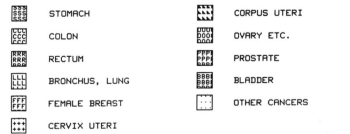

STOMACH	CORPUS UTERI
COLON	OVARY ETC.
RECTUM	PROSTATE
BRONCHUS, LUNG	BLADDER
FEMALE BREAST	OTHER CANCERS
CERVIX UTERI	

FRANCE, BAS-RHIN

M

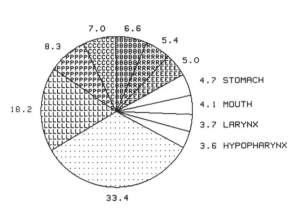

7.0 6.6
8.3 5.4
5.0
4.7 STOMACH
4.1 MOUTH
3.7 LARYNX
3.6 HYPOPHARYNX
18.2
33.4

F

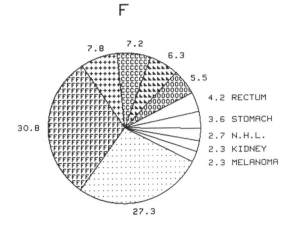

7.8 7.2
6.3
5.5
4.2 RECTUM
3.6 STOMACH
2.7 N.H.L.
2.3 KIDNEY
2.3 MELANOMA
30.8
27.3

FRANCE, CALVADOS

M

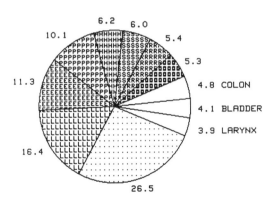

6.2 6.0
10.1 5.4
5.3
4.8 COLON
4.1 BLADDER
3.9 LARYNX
11.3
16.4
26.5

F

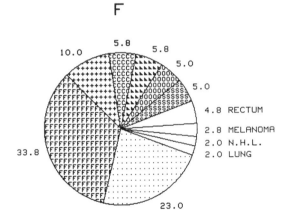

5.8 5.8
10.0 5.0
5.0
4.8 RECTUM
2.8 MELANOMA
2.0 N.H.L.
2.0 LUNG
33.8
23.0

FRANCE, DOUBS

M

6.5 6.2
8.8 6.2
5.4
4.5 LARYNX
4.3 OESOPHAGUS
3.1 HYPOPHARYNX
3.0 OROPHARYNX
18.0
34.0

F

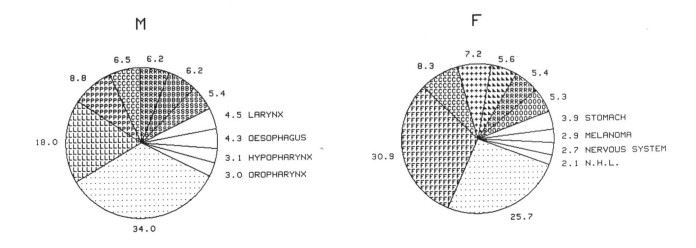

7.2 5.6
8.3 5.4
5.3
3.9 STOMACH
2.9 MELANOMA
2.7 NERVOUS SYSTEM
2.1 N.H.L.
30.9
25.7

FRANCE, ISERE

M

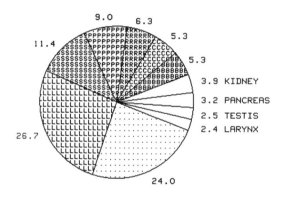

9.6
6.6
6.2
5.3
4.8 LARYNX
4.7 STOMACH
4.2 OESOPHAGUS
2.8 KIDNEY
2.6 N.H.L.
18.4
34.8

F

7.7
7.6
5.7
4.9 RECTUM
4.7 OVARY
3.2 STOMACH
2.6 NERVOUS SYSTEM
2.5 N.H.L.
2.3 LUNG
34.3
24.5

GERMAN DEMOCRATIC REPUBLIC

M

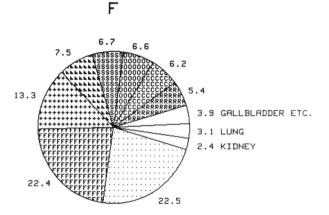

9.0
6.3
5.3
5.3
3.9 KIDNEY
3.2 PANCREAS
2.5 TESTIS
2.4 LARYNX
11.4
26.7
24.0

F

6.7
6.6
7.5
6.2
5.4
13.3
3.9 GALLBLADDER ETC.
3.1 LUNG
2.4 KIDNEY
22.4
22.5

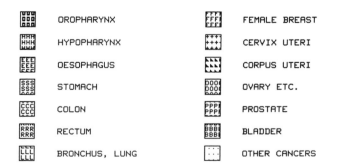

OROPHARYNX	FEMALE BREAST
HYPOPHARYNX	CERVIX UTERI
OESOPHAGUS	CORPUS UTERI
STOMACH	OVARY ETC.
COLON	PROSTATE
RECTUM	BLADDER
BRONCHUS, LUNG	OTHER CANCERS

HUNGARY, COUNTY SZABOLCS-SZATMAR

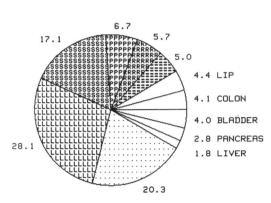

M

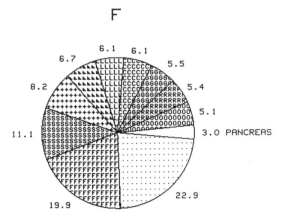

F

HUNGARY, COUNTY VAS

M

F

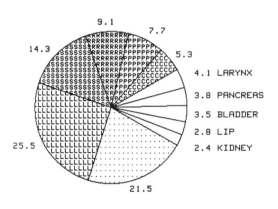

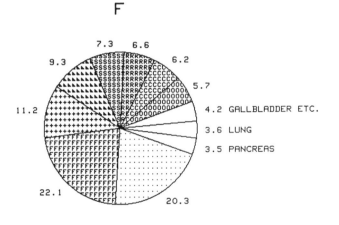

ICELAND

M

F

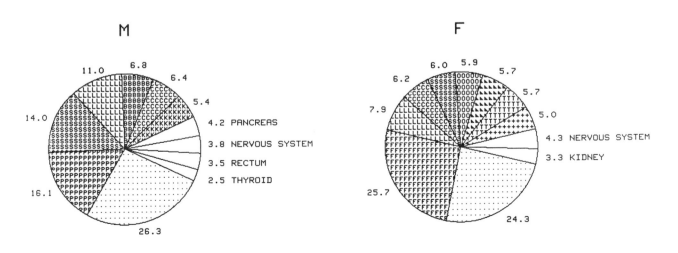

IRELAND, SOUTHERN

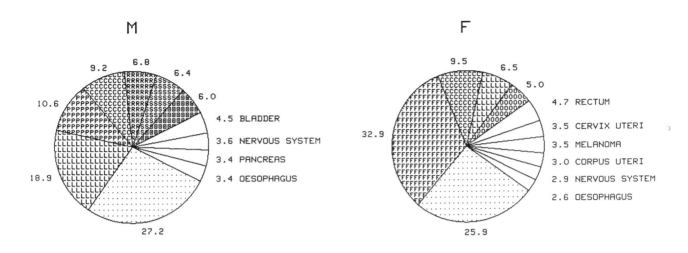

M

9.2 6.8 6.4
10.6 6.0
18.9 4.5 BLADDER
3.6 NERVOUS SYSTEM
3.4 PANCREAS
3.4 OESOPHAGUS
27.2

F

9.5 6.5
5.0
4.7 RECTUM
3.5 CERVIX UTERI
32.9 3.5 MELANOMA
3.0 CORPUS UTERI
2.9 NERVOUS SYSTEM
2.6 OESOPHAGUS
25.9

ITALY, LOMBARDY REGION, VARESE PROVINCE

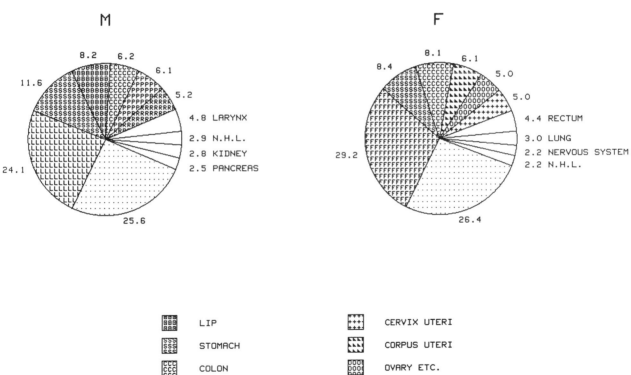

M

8.2 6.2
11.6 6.1
5.2
4.8 LARYNX
2.9 N.H.L.
24.1 2.8 KIDNEY
2.5 PANCREAS
25.6

F

8.1 6.1
8.4 5.0
5.0
4.4 RECTUM
3.0 LUNG
29.2 2.2 NERVOUS SYSTEM
2.2 N.H.L.
26.4

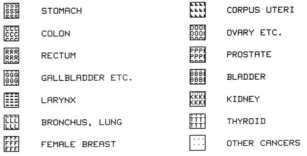

LIP   CERVIX UTERI

STOMACH   CORPUS UTERI

COLON   OVARY ETC.

RECTUM   PROSTATE

GALLBLADDER ETC.   BLADDER

LARYNX   KIDNEY

BRONCHUS, LUNG   THYROID

FEMALE BREAST   OTHER CANCERS

ITALY, PARMA PROVINCE

M

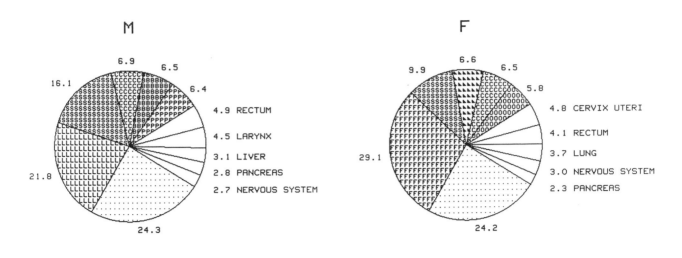

6.9 6.5
16.1 6.4
4.9 RECTUM
4.5 LARYNX
3.1 LIVER
2.8 PANCREAS
2.7 NERVOUS SYSTEM
21.8
24.3

F

6.6 6.5
9.9 5.8
4.8 CERVIX UTERI
4.1 RECTUM
3.7 LUNG
3.0 NERVOUS SYSTEM
2.3 PANCREAS
29.1
24.2

ITALY, RAGUSA PROVINCE

M

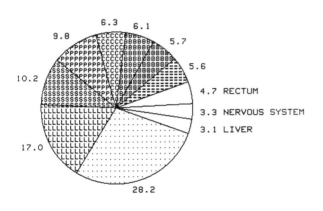

6.3 6.1
9.8 5.7
5.6
4.7 RECTUM
3.3 NERVOUS SYSTEM
3.1 LIVER
10.2
17.0
28.2

F

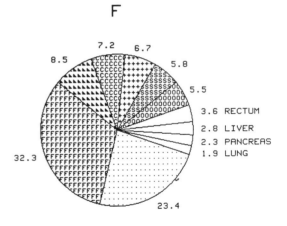

7.2 6.7
8.5 5.8
5.5
3.6 RECTUM
2.8 LIVER
2.3 PANCREAS
1.9 LUNG
32.3
23.4

NETHERLANDS, EINDHOVEN

M

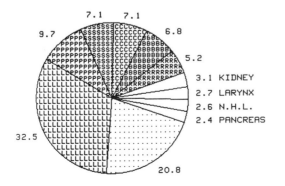

7.1 7.1
9.7 6.8
5.2
3.1 KIDNEY
2.7 LARYNX
2.6 N.H.L.
2.4 PANCREAS
32.5
20.8

F

9.7 5.7
5.1
4.6 STOMACH
4.4 RECTUM
3.7 CERVIX UTERI
2.9 MELANOMA
2.8 LUNG
2.1 KIDNEY
35.1
23.9

NORWAY

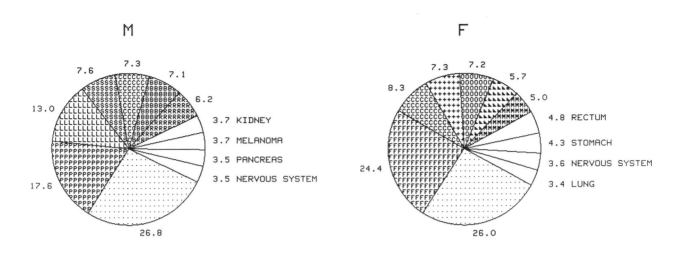

M

7.6 7.3 7.1
6.2
13.0
3.7 KIDNEY
3.7 MELANOMA
3.5 PANCREAS
17.6
3.5 NERVOUS SYSTEM
26.8

F

7.3 7.2 5.7
8.3
5.0
4.8 RECTUM
4.3 STOMACH
3.6 NERVOUS SYSTEM
24.4
3.4 LUNG
26.0

POLAND, CRACOW CITY

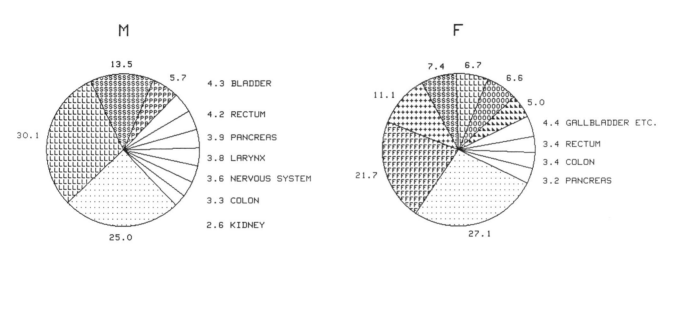

M

13.5
5.7
4.3 BLADDER
4.2 RECTUM
3.9 PANCREAS
30.1
3.8 LARYNX
3.6 NERVOUS SYSTEM
3.3 COLON
2.6 KIDNEY
25.0

F

7.4 6.7 6.6
11.1
5.0
4.4 GALLBLADDER ETC.
3.4 RECTUM
3.4 COLON
21.7
3.2 PANCREAS
27.1

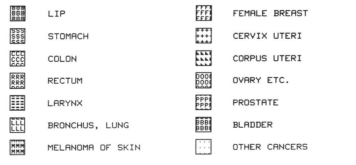

LIP

STOMACH

COLON

RECTUM

LARYNX

BRONCHUS, LUNG

MELANOMA OF SKIN

FEMALE BREAST

CERVIX UTERI

CORPUS UTERI

OVARY ETC.

PROSTATE

BLADDER

OTHER CANCERS

POLAND, NOWY SACZ RURAL AREAS

M

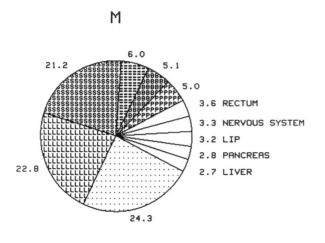

21.2 6.0 5.1

5.0

3.6 RECTUM
3.3 NERVOUS SYSTEM
3.2 LIP
2.8 PANCREAS
2.7 LIVER

22.8

24.3

F

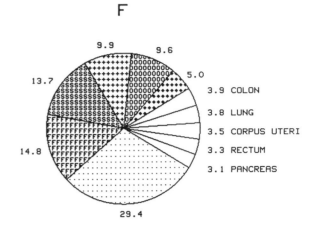

9.9 9.6

13.7

5.0

3.9 COLON
3.8 LUNG
3.5 CORPUS UTERI
3.3 RECTUM
3.1 PANCREAS

14.8

29.4

POLAND, WARSAW CITY

M

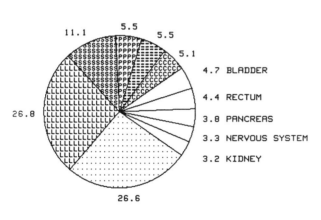

11.1 5.5 5.5

5.1

4.7 BLADDER
4.4 RECTUM
3.8 PANCREAS
3.3 NERVOUS SYSTEM
3.2 KIDNEY

26.8

26.6

F

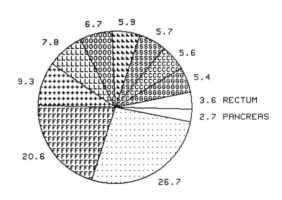

6.7 5.9 5.7

7.8

5.6

9.3

5.4

3.6 RECTUM
2.7 PANCREAS

20.6

26.7

ROMANIA, COUNTY CLUJ

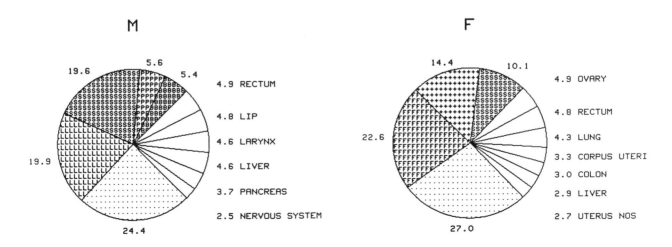

M

19.6 5.6 5.4

4.9 RECTUM
4.8 LIP
4.6 LARYNX
4.6 LIVER
3.7 PANCREAS
2.5 NERVOUS SYSTEM

19.9

24.4

F

14.4 10.1

22.6

4.9 OVARY
4.8 RECTUM
4.3 LUNG
3.3 CORPUS UTERI
3.0 COLON
2.9 LIVER
2.7 UTERUS NOS

27.0

SPAIN, CATALONIA, TARRAGONA

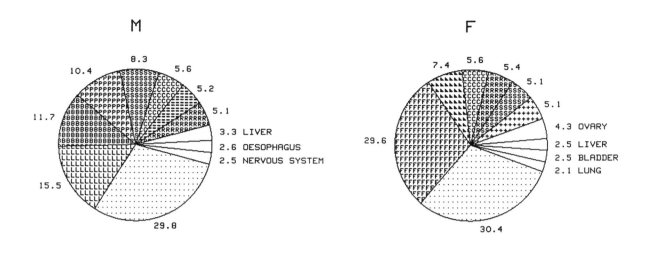

M

8.3
10.4
5.6
5.2
11.7
5.1
3.3 LIVER
2.6 OESOPHAGUS
2.5 NERVOUS SYSTEM
15.5
29.8

F

7.4
5.6
5.4
5.1
5.1
4.3 OVARY
2.5 LIVER
2.5 BLADDER
2.1 LUNG
29.6
30.4

SPAIN, NAVARRA

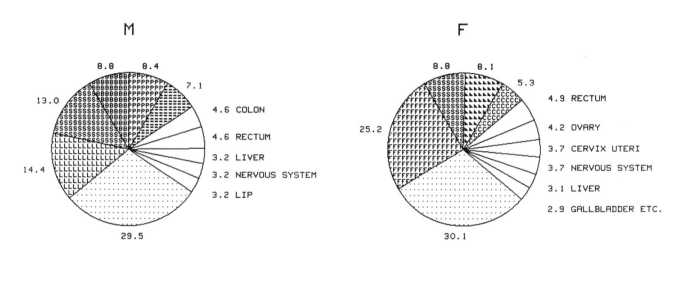

M

8.8
8.4
7.1
13.0
4.6 COLON
4.6 RECTUM
3.2 LIVER
14.4
3.2 NERVOUS SYSTEM
3.2 LIP
29.5

F

8.8
8.1
5.3
4.9 RECTUM
25.2
4.2 OVARY
3.7 CERVIX UTERI
3.7 NERVOUS SYSTEM
3.1 LIVER
2.9 GALLBLADDER ETC.
30.1

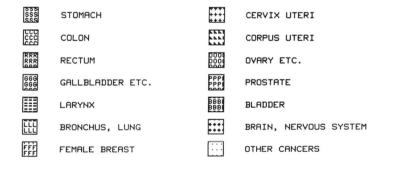

SSS	STOMACH	+++	CERVIX UTERI
CCC	COLON	\\\	CORPUS UTERI
RRR	RECTUM	OOO	OVARY ETC.
GGG	GALLBLADDER ETC.	PPP	PROSTATE
⊞	LARYNX	BBB	BLADDER
LLL	BRONCHUS, LUNG	•••	BRAIN, NERVOUS SYSTEM
FFF	FEMALE BREAST	⋮	OTHER CANCERS

SPAIN, ZARAGOZA

M

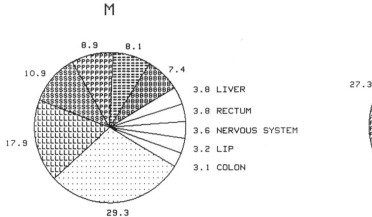

8.9   8.1   7.4

10.9

17.9

29.3

3.8 LIVER
3.8 RECTUM
3.6 NERVOUS SYSTEM
3.2 LIP
3.1 COLON

F

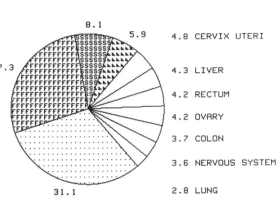

8.1   5.9

27.3

31.1

4.8 CERVIX UTERI
4.3 LIVER
4.2 RECTUM
4.2 OVARY
3.7 COLON
3.6 NERVOUS SYSTEM
2.8 LUNG

SWEDEN

M

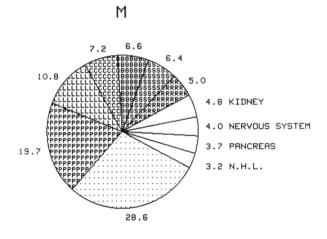

7.2   6.6   6.4

10.8

19.7

28.6

5.0

4.8 KIDNEY
4.0 NERVOUS SYSTEM
3.7 PANCREAS
3.2 N.H.L.

F

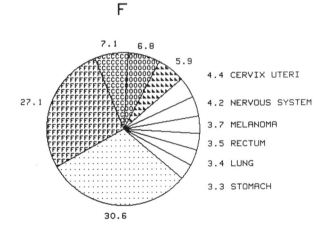

7.1   6.8

27.1

30.6

5.9

4.4 CERVIX UTERI
4.2 NERVOUS SYSTEM
3.7 MELANOMA
3.5 RECTUM
3.4 LUNG
3.3 STOMACH

SWITZERLAND, BASEL

M

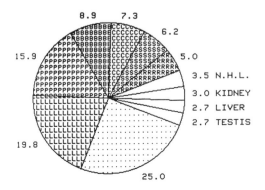

8.9   7.3

15.9

19.8

25.0

6.2

5.0

3.5 N.H.L.
3.0 KIDNEY
2.7 LIVER
2.7 TESTIS

F

7.1   6.7

33.2

27.0

4.5 OVARY
4.3 RECTUM
4.0 STOMACH
3.8 LUNG
3.2 CERVIX UTERI
3.1 MELANOMA
3.1 KIDNEY

SWITZERLAND, GENEVA

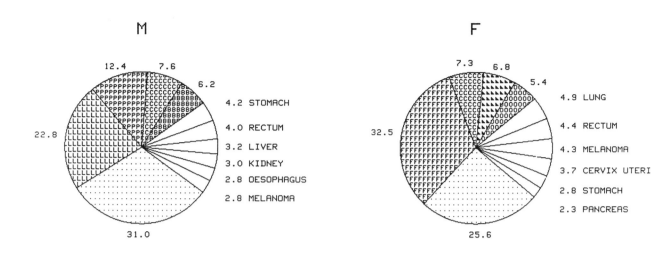

M

12.4 7.6
6.2
4.2 STOMACH
4.0 RECTUM
3.2 LIVER
3.0 KIDNEY
2.8 OESOPHAGUS
2.8 MELANOMA
22.8
31.0

F

7.3 6.8
5.4
4.9 LUNG
4.4 RECTUM
4.3 MELANOMA
3.7 CERVIX UTERI
2.8 STOMACH
2.3 PANCREAS
32.5
25.6

SWITZERLAND, NEUCHATEL

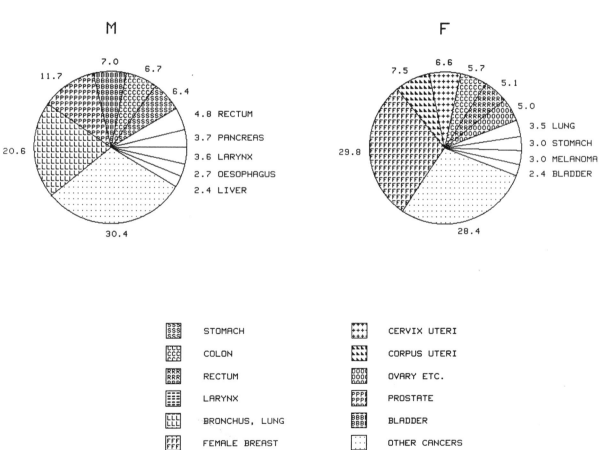

M

7.0 6.7
11.7
6.4
4.8 RECTUM
3.7 PANCREAS
3.6 LARYNX
2.7 OESOPHAGUS
2.4 LIVER
20.6
30.4

F

6.6
7.5 5.7
5.1
5.0
3.5 LUNG
3.0 STOMACH
3.0 MELANOMA
2.4 BLADDER
29.8
28.4

STOMACH	CERVIX UTERI	
COLON	CORPUS UTERI	
RECTUM	OVARY ETC.	
LARYNX	PROSTATE	
BRONCHUS, LUNG	BLADDER	
FEMALE BREAST	OTHER CANCERS	

97

SWITZERLAND, VAUD

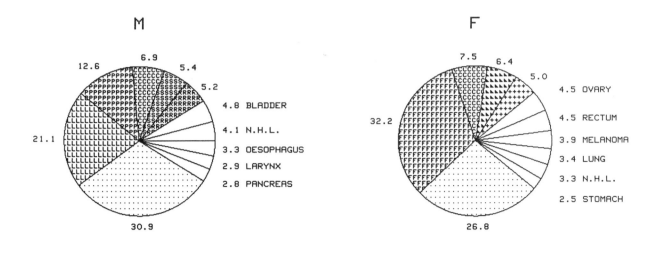

M

12.6   6.9   5.4

5.2

21.1

4.8 BLADDER

4.1 N.H.L.

3.3 OESOPHAGUS

2.9 LARYNX

2.8 PANCREAS

30.9

F

7.5   6.4

5.0

32.2

4.5 OVARY

4.5 RECTUM

3.9 MELANOMA

3.4 LUNG

3.3 N.H.L.

2.5 STOMACH

26.8

SWITZERLAND, ZURICH

M

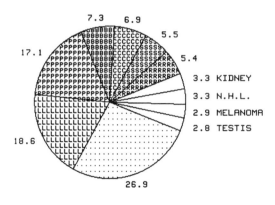

7.3   6.9

5.5

17.1

5.4

3.3 KIDNEY

3.3 N.H.L.

2.9 MELANOMA

2.8 TESTIS

18.6

26.9

F

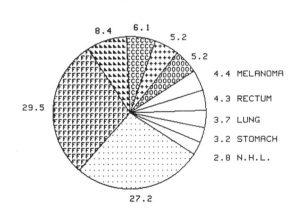

8.4   6.1

5.2

5.2

29.5

4.4 MELANOMA

4.3 RECTUM

3.7 LUNG

3.2 STOMACH

2.8 N.H.L.

27.2

UK, ENGLAND AND WALES

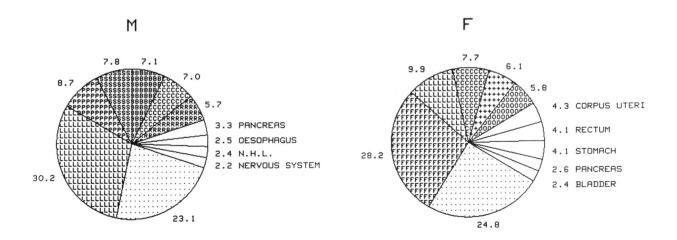

M

7.8   7.1

7.0

8.7

5.7

3.3 PANCREAS

2.5 OESOPHAGUS

2.4 N.H.L.

2.2 NERVOUS SYSTEM

30.2

23.1

F

9.9   7.7   6.1

5.8

28.2

4.3 CORPUS UTERI

4.1 RECTUM

4.1 STOMACH

2.6 PANCREAS

2.4 BLADDER

24.8

UK, BIRMINGHAM AND WEST MIDLANDS REGION

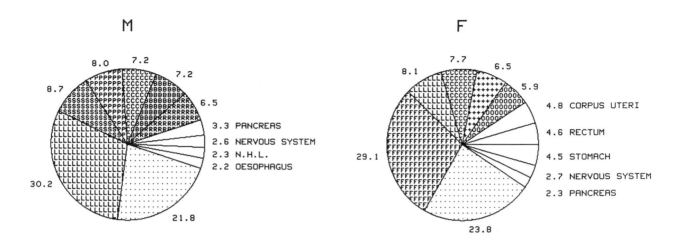

M

8.0   7.2
7.2
8.7
6.5

3.3 PANCREAS
2.6 NERVOUS SYSTEM
2.3 N.H.L.
2.2 OESOPHAGUS

30.2

21.8

F

7.7   6.5
8.1
5.9

4.8 CORPUS UTERI
4.6 RECTUM
4.5 STOMACH
2.7 NERVOUS SYSTEM
2.3 PANCREAS

29.1

23.8

UK, ENGLAND, NORTH WESTERN REGION

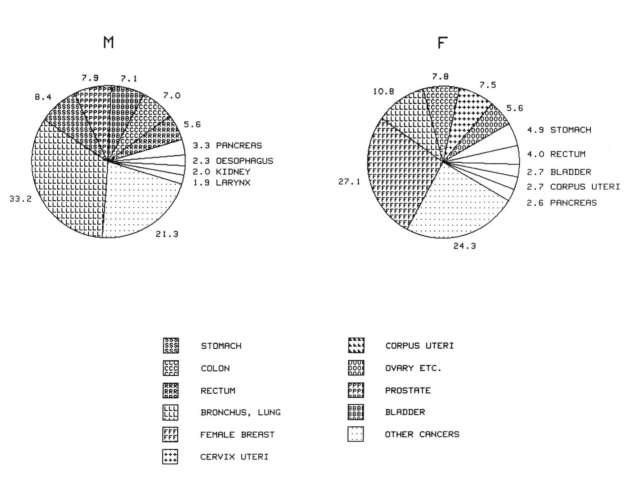

M

7.9   7.1
8.4
7.0
5.6

3.3 PANCREAS
2.3 OESOPHAGUS
2.0 KIDNEY
1.9 LARYNX

33.2

21.3

F

7.8   7.5
10.8
5.6

4.9 STOMACH
4.0 RECTUM
2.7 BLADDER
2.7 CORPUS UTERI
2.6 PANCREAS

27.1

24.3

STOMACH		CORPUS UTERI
COLON		OVARY ETC.
RECTUM		PROSTATE
BRONCHUS, LUNG		BLADDER
FEMALE BREAST		OTHER CANCERS
CERVIX UTERI		

UK, ENGLAND, OXFORD REGION

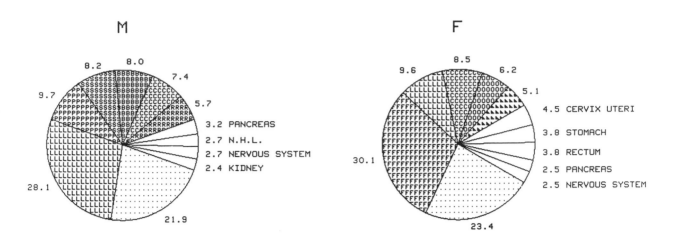

M

F

8.2 8.0 7.4 9.7 5.7 28.1 21.9

3.2 PANCREAS
2.7 N.H.L.
2.7 NERVOUS SYSTEM
2.4 KIDNEY

8.5 9.6 6.2 5.1 30.1 23.4

4.5 CERVIX UTERI
3.8 STOMACH
3.8 RECTUM
2.5 PANCREAS
2.5 NERVOUS SYSTEM

UK, ENGLAND, SOUTH THAMES REGION

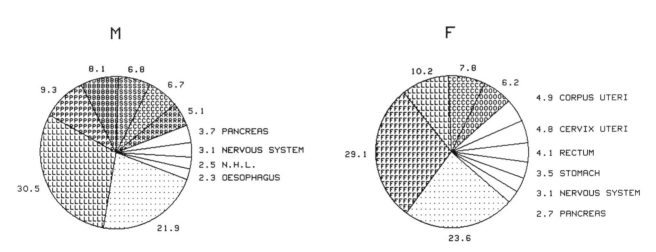

M

F

8.1 6.8 6.7 9.3 5.1 30.5 21.9

3.7 PANCREAS
3.1 NERVOUS SYSTEM
2.5 N.H.L.
2.3 OESOPHAGUS

10.2 7.8 6.2 29.1 23.6

4.9 CORPUS UTERI
4.8 CERVIX UTERI
4.1 RECTUM
3.5 STOMACH
3.1 NERVOUS SYSTEM
2.7 PANCREAS

UK, ENGLAND, SOUTH WESTERN REGION

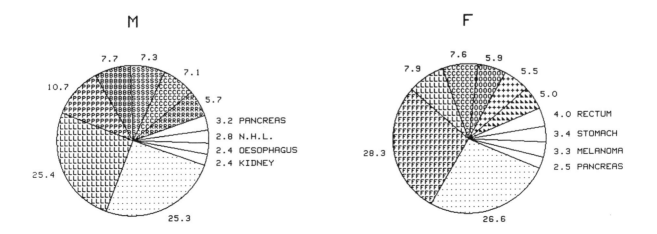

M

F

7.7 7.3 7.1 10.7 5.7 25.4 25.3

3.2 PANCREAS
2.8 N.H.L.
2.4 OESOPHAGUS
2.4 KIDNEY

7.6 5.9 7.9 5.5 5.0 28.3 26.6

4.0 RECTUM
3.4 STOMACH
3.3 MELANOMA
2.5 PANCREAS

UK, ENGLAND, TRENT REGION

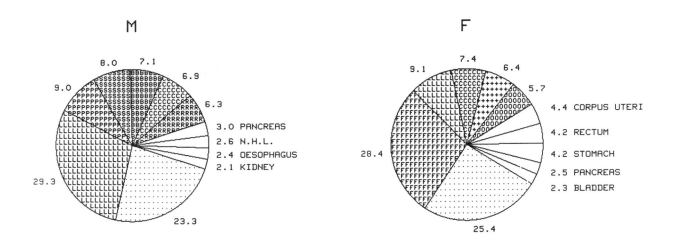

M

8.0 7.1
9.0 6.9
6.3
3.0 PANCREAS
2.6 N.H.L.
2.4 OESOPHAGUS
2.1 KIDNEY
29.3
23.3

F

7.4 6.4
9.1 5.7
4.4 CORPUS UTERI
4.2 RECTUM
4.2 STOMACH
2.5 PANCREAS
2.3 BLADDER
28.4
25.4

UK, ENGLAND AND WALES, MERSEY REGION

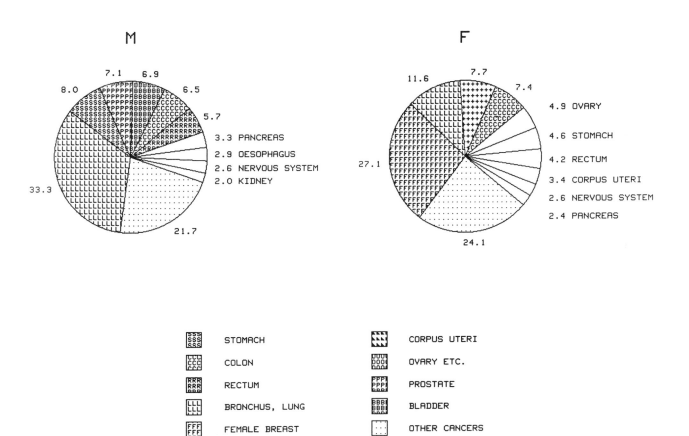

M

7.1 6.9
8.0 6.5
5.7
3.3 PANCREAS
2.9 OESOPHAGUS
2.6 NERVOUS SYSTEM
2.0 KIDNEY
33.3
21.7

F

7.7 7.4
11.6
4.9 OVARY
4.6 STOMACH
4.2 RECTUM
3.4 CORPUS UTERI
2.6 NERVOUS SYSTEM
2.4 PANCREAS
27.1
24.1

- STOMACH
- COLON
- RECTUM
- BRONCHUS, LUNG
- FEMALE BREAST
- CERVIX UTERI
- CORPUS UTERI
- OVARY ETC.
- PROSTATE
- BLADDER
- OTHER CANCERS

UK, SCOTLAND

M

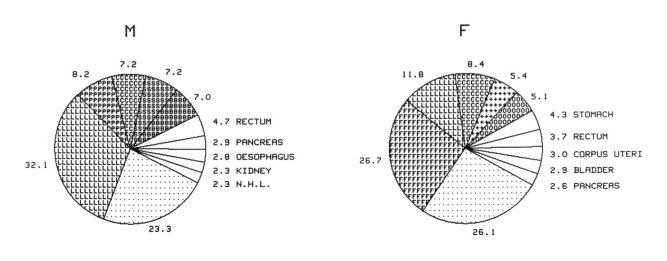

```
7.2
8.2        7.2
                   7.0
                   4.7 RECTUM
                   2.9 PANCREAS
                   2.8 OESOPHAGUS
                   2.3 KIDNEY
32.1               2.3 N.H.L.

        23.3
```

F

```
8.4
11.8       5.4
                   5.1
                   4.3 STOMACH
                   3.7 RECTUM
                   3.0 CORPUS UTERI
                   2.9 BLADDER
26.7               2.6 PANCREAS

        26.1
```

UK, SCOTLAND, EAST

M

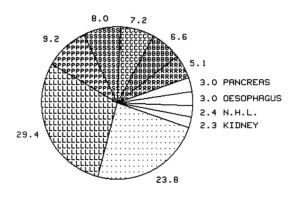

```
8.0    7.2
9.2            6.6
                   5.1
                   3.0 PANCREAS
                   3.0 OESOPHAGUS
                   2.4 N.H.L.
29.4               2.3 KIDNEY

        23.8
```

F

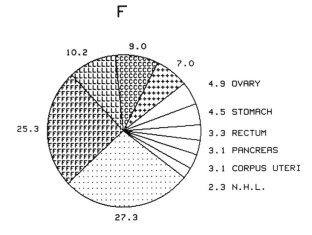

```
9.0
10.2           7.0
                   4.9 OVARY
                   4.5 STOMACH
                   3.3 RECTUM
                   3.1 PANCREAS
25.3               3.1 CORPUS UTERI
                   2.3 N.H.L.

        27.3
```

UK, SCOTLAND, NORTH

M

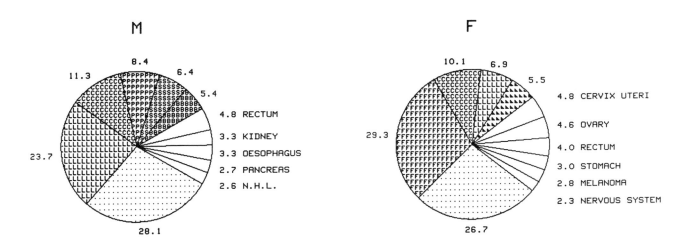

```
8.4
11.3       6.4
                   5.4
                   4.8 RECTUM
                   3.3 KIDNEY
                   3.3 OESOPHAGUS
23.7               2.7 PANCREAS
                   2.6 N.H.L.

        28.1
```

F

```
10.1   6.9
                   5.5
                   4.8 CERVIX UTERI
                   4.6 OVARY
                   4.0 RECTUM
29.3               3.0 STOMACH
                   2.8 MELANOMA
                   2.3 NERVOUS SYSTEM

        26.7
```

UK, SCOTLAND, NORTH-EAST

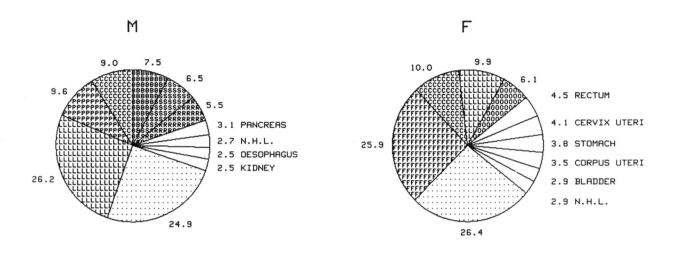

UK, SCOTLAND, SOUTH-EAST

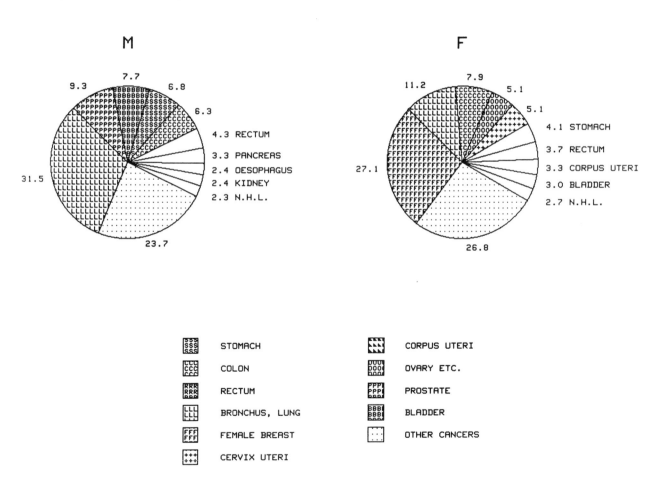

UK, SCOTLAND, WEST

M

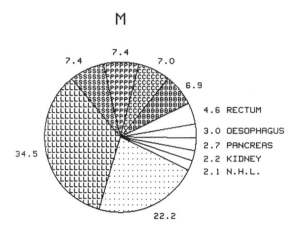

```
7.4        7.4     7.0
      7.4
                      6.9
                            4.6 RECTUM
                            3.0 OESOPHAGUS
                            2.7 PANCREAS
34.5                        2.2 KIDNEY
                            2.1 N.H.L.

           22.2
```

F

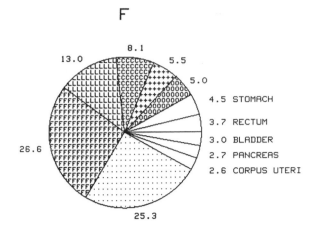

```
          8.1
13.0              5.5
                       5.0
                            4.5 STOMACH
                            3.7 RECTUM
                            3.0 BLADDER
26.6                        2.7 PANCREAS
                            2.6 CORPUS UTERI

           25.3
```

YUGOSLAVIA, SLOVENIA

M

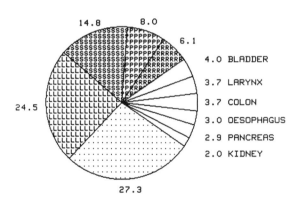

```
14.8      8.0
               6.1
                    4.0 BLADDER
                    3.7 LARYNX
                    3.7 COLON
24.5                3.0 OESOPHAGUS
                    2.9 PANCREAS
                    2.0 KIDNEY

      27.3
```

F

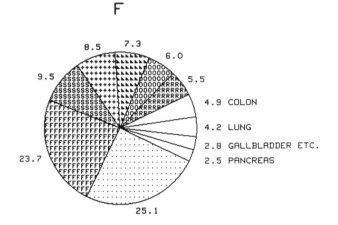

```
    8.5   7.3
                6.0
9.5                 5.5
                         4.9 COLON
                         4.2 LUNG
                         2.8 GALLBLADDER ETC.
23.7                     2.5 PANCREAS

           25.1
```

AUSTRALIAN CAPITAL TERRITORY

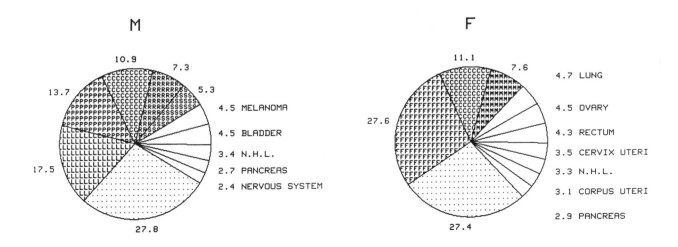

M

```
      10.9    7.3
13.7               5.3
                        4.5 MELANOMA
                        4.5 BLADDER
                        3.4 N.H.L.
17.5                    2.7 PANCREAS
                        2.4 NERVOUS SYSTEM

           27.8
```

F

```
      11.1    7.6
                        4.7 LUNG
                        4.5 OVARY
27.6                    4.3 RECTUM
                        3.5 CERVIX UTERI
                        3.3 N.H.L.
                        3.1 CORPUS UTERI

                        2.9 PANCREAS
           27.4
```

AUSTRALIA, NEW SOUTH WALES

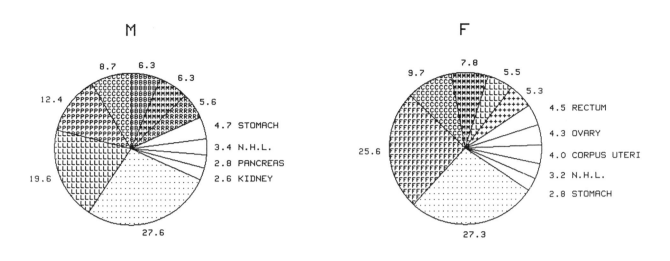

M

8.7   6.3
6.3
12.4   5.6
                        4.7 STOMACH
                        3.4 N.H.L.
                        2.8 PANCREAS
                        2.6 KIDNEY
19.6
27.6

F

7.8
9.7   5.5
                5.3
                4.5 RECTUM
                4.3 OVARY
                4.0 CORPUS UTERI
                3.2 N.H.L.
25.6   2.8 STOMACH
27.3

AUSTRALIA, QUEENSLAND

M

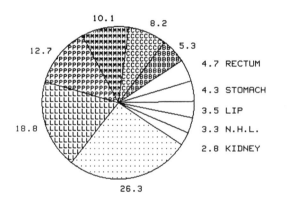

10.1   8.2
12.7   5.3
                4.7 RECTUM
                4.3 STOMACH
                3.5 LIP
                3.3 N.H.L.
                2.8 KIDNEY
18.8
26.3

F

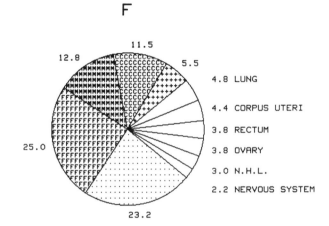

11.5
12.8   5.5
                4.8 LUNG
                4.4 CORPUS UTERI
                3.8 RECTUM
                3.8 OVARY
                3.0 N.H.L.
25.0   2.2 NERVOUS SYSTEM
23.2

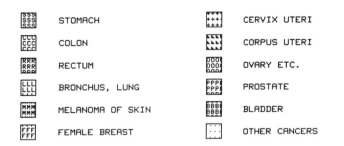

STOMACH   CERVIX UTERI

COLON   CORPUS UTERI

RECTUM   OVARY ETC.

BRONCHUS, LUNG   PROSTATE

MELANOMA OF SKIN   BLADDER

FEMALE BREAST   OTHER CANCERS

105

SOUTH AUSTRALIA

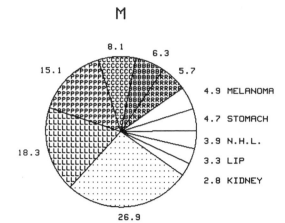

M

8.1 6.3
15.1 5.7
4.9 MELANOMA
4.7 STOMACH
3.9 N.H.L.
18.3 3.3 LIP
2.8 KIDNEY
26.9

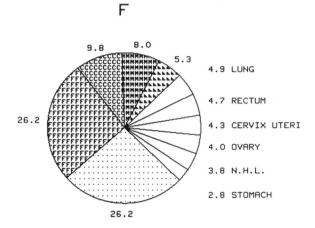

F

9.8 8.0
5.3
4.9 LUNG
4.7 RECTUM
26.2 4.3 CERVIX UTERI
4.0 OVARY
3.8 N.H.L.
2.8 STOMACH
26.2

AUSTRALIA, TASMANIA

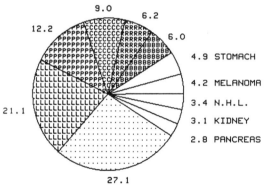
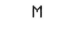

M

9.0 6.2
12.2 6.0
4.9 STOMACH
4.2 MELANOMA
3.4 N.H.L.
21.1 3.1 KIDNEY
2.8 PANCREAS
27.1

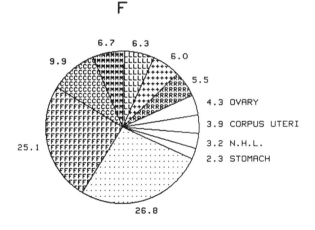

F

6.7 6.3
9.9 6.0
5.5
4.3 OVARY
3.9 CORPUS UTERI
25.1 3.2 N.H.L.
2.3 STOMACH
26.8

AUSTRALIA, VICTORIA

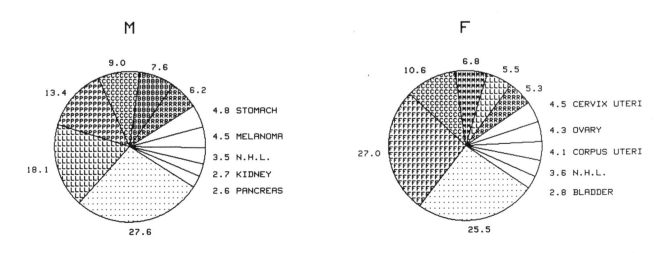

M

9.0 7.6
13.4 6.2
4.8 STOMACH
4.5 MELANOMA
3.5 N.H.L.
18.1 2.7 KIDNEY
2.6 PANCREAS
27.6

F

6.8 5.5
10.6 5.3
4.5 CERVIX UTERI
4.3 OVARY
27.0 4.1 CORPUS UTERI
3.6 N.H.L.
2.8 BLADDER
25.5

WESTERN AUSTRALIA

M

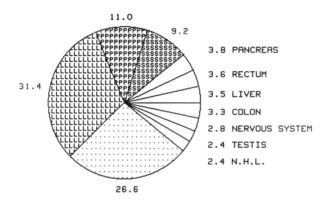

7.9 6.8 8.0 5.7 12.0 5.5 3.6 N.H.L. 2.5 KIDNEY 2.2 PANCREAS 19.5 26.3

F

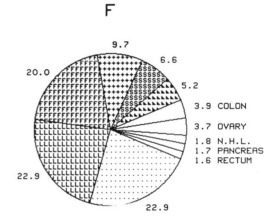

8.0 6.7 10.3 6.3 4.7 CORPUS UTERI 4.6 RECTUM 4.2 OVARY 3.4 N.H.L. 2.8 BLADDER 25.1 23.9

NEW ZEALAND: MAORI

M

11.0 9.2 3.8 PANCREAS 3.6 RECTUM 3.5 LIVER 3.3 COLON 2.8 NERVOUS SYSTEM 2.4 TESTIS 2.4 N.H.L. 31.4 26.6

F

9.7 6.6 20.0 5.2 3.9 COLON 3.7 OVARY 1.8 N.H.L. 1.7 PANCREAS 1.6 RECTUM 22.9 22.9

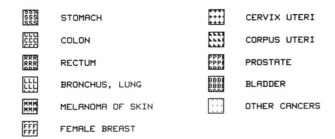

	STOMACH		CERVIX UTERI
	COLON		CORPUS UTERI
	RECTUM		PROSTATE
	BRONCHUS, LUNG		BLADDER
	MELANOMA OF SKIN		OTHER CANCERS
	FEMALE BREAST		

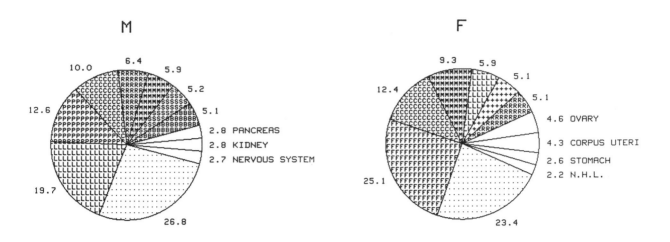

NEW ZEALAND: NON-MAORI

M

10.0 6.4 5.9
12.6   5.2
    5.1
2.8 PANCREAS
2.8 KIDNEY
2.7 NERVOUS SYSTEM
19.7
26.8

F

9.3 5.9
12.4   5.1
    5.1
4.6 OVARY
4.3 CORPUS UTERI
2.6 STOMACH
2.2 N.H.L.
25.1
23.4

NEW ZEALAND: PACIFIC POLYNESIAN ISLANDERS

M

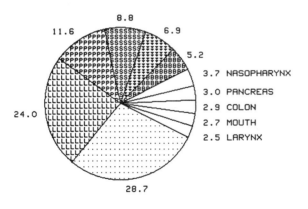

8.8 6.9
11.6   5.2
3.7 NASOPHARYNX
3.0 PANCREAS
2.9 COLON
2.7 MOUTH
2.5 LARYNX
24.0
28.7

F

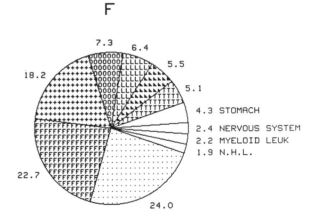

7.3 6.4
18.2   5.5
    5.1
4.3 STOMACH
2.4 NERVOUS SYSTEM
2.2 MYELOID LEUK
1.9 N.H.L.
22.7
24.0

USA, HAWAII: WHITE

M

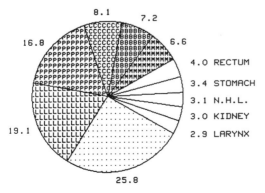

8.1 7.2
16.8   6.6
4.0 RECTUM
3.4 STOMACH
3.1 N.H.L.
3.0 KIDNEY
2.9 LARYNX
19.1
25.8

F

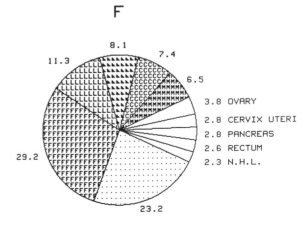

8.1 7.4
11.3   6.5
3.8 OVARY
2.8 CERVIX UTERI
2.8 PANCREAS
2.6 RECTUM
2.3 N.H.L.
29.2
23.2

USA, HAWAII: JAPANESE

M

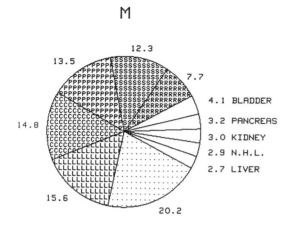

12.3
13.5
7.7
14.8
15.6
20.2

4.1 BLADDER
3.2 PANCREAS
3.0 KIDNEY
2.9 N.H.L.
2.7 LIVER

F

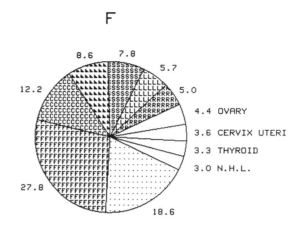

8.6   7.8
5.7
12.2
5.0
27.8
18.6

4.4 OVARY
3.6 CERVIX UTERI
3.3 THYROID
3.0 N.H.L.

USA, HAWAII: HAWAIIAN

M

10.0
6.4
13.1
5.2
26.6
23.3

3.5 OESOPHAGUS
3.2 N.H.L.
3.2 BLADDER
2.9 PANCREAS
2.6 KIDNEY

F

13.3   8.5
5.0
31.6
20.4

4.7 OVARY
4.1 CERVIX UTERI
4.0 COLON
3.5 THYROID
2.6 PANCREAS
2.3 RECTUM

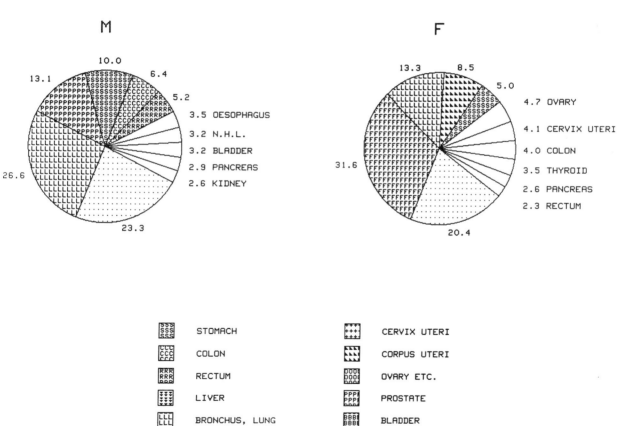

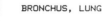

STOMACH		CERVIX UTERI
COLON		CORPUS UTERI
RECTUM		OVARY ETC.
LIVER		PROSTATE
BRONCHUS, LUNG		BLADDER
MELANOMA OF SKIN		THYROID
FEMALE BREAST		OTHER CANCERS

USA, HAWAII: FILIPINO

M

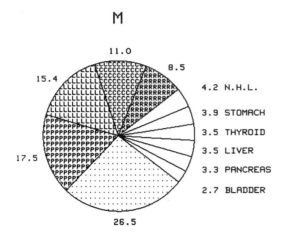

11.0
8.5
15.4
4.2 N.H.L.
3.9 STOMACH
3.5 THYROID
3.5 LIVER
3.3 PANCREAS
17.5
2.7 BLADDER
26.5

F

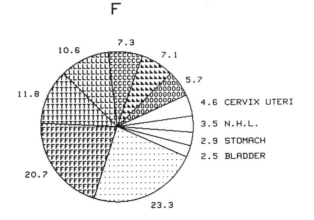

7.3
10.6
7.1
5.7
11.8
4.6 CERVIX UTERI
3.5 N.H.L.
2.9 STOMACH
2.5 BLADDER
20.7
23.3

USA, HAWAII: CHINESE

M

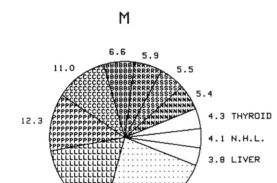

6.6   5.9
11.0
5.5
5.4
12.3
4.3 THYROID
4.1 N.H.L.
3.8 LIVER
17.9
23.2

F

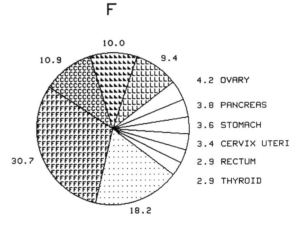

10.0
10.9   9.4
4.2 OVARY
3.8 PANCREAS
3.6 STOMACH
3.4 CERVIX UTERI
2.9 RECTUM
2.9 THYROID
30.7
18.2

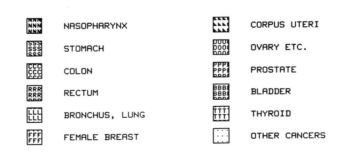

NASOPHARYNX		CORPUS UTERI	
STOMACH		OVARY ETC.	
COLON		PROSTATE	
RECTUM		BLADDER	
BRONCHUS, LUNG		THYROID	
FEMALE BREAST		OTHER CANCERS	

Part III

Graphs of age-specific cancer incidence rates by site and sex

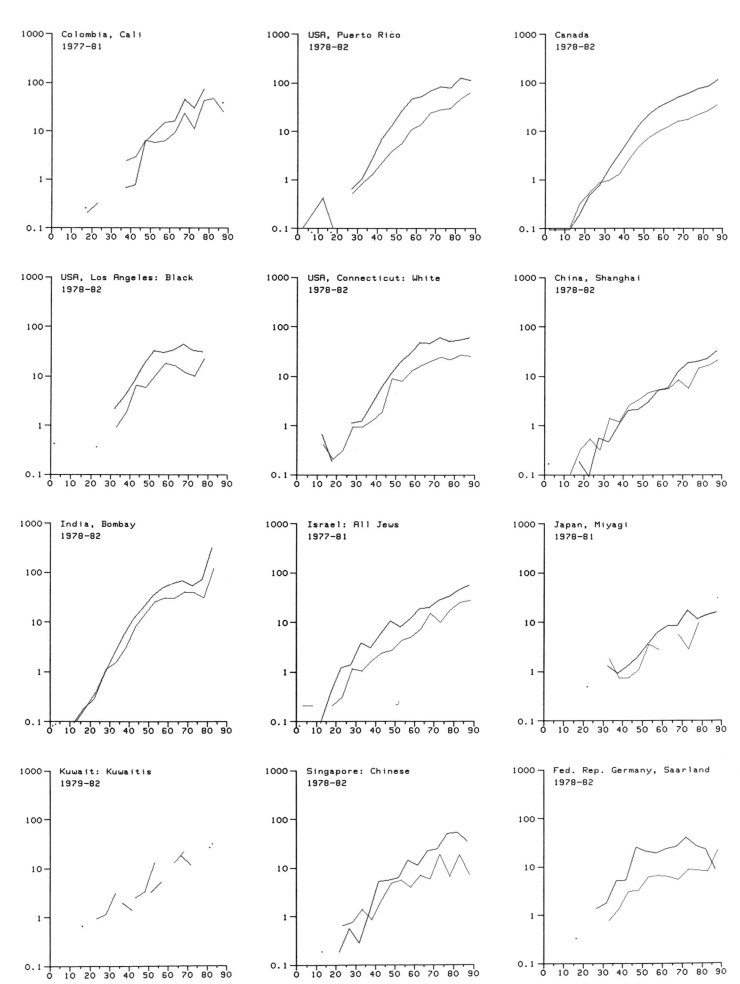

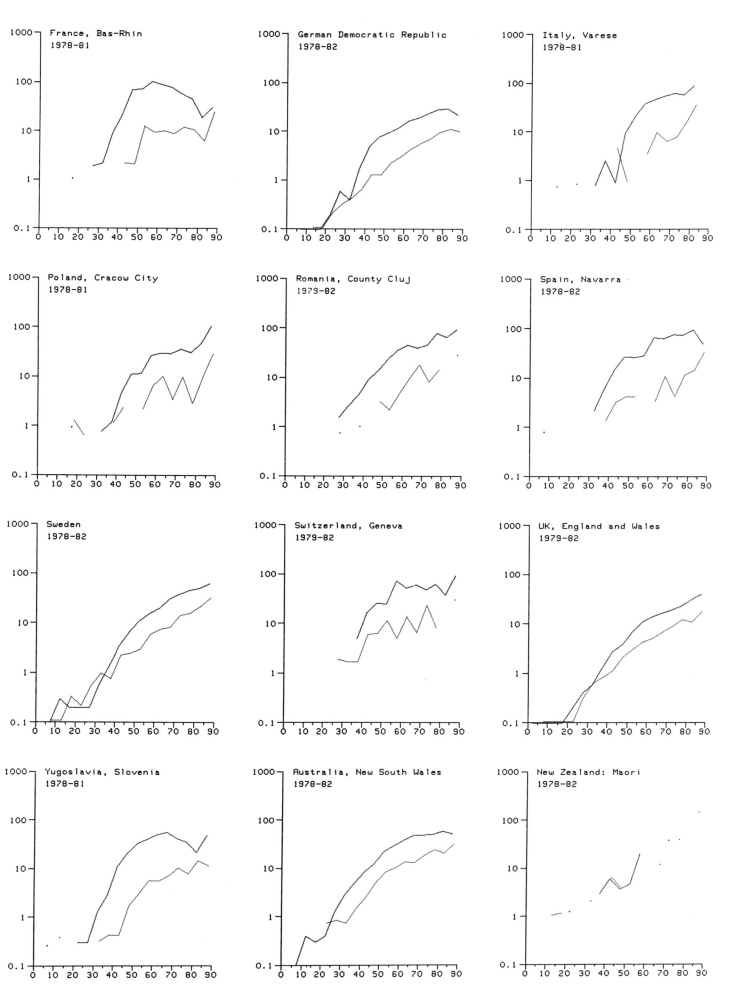

113

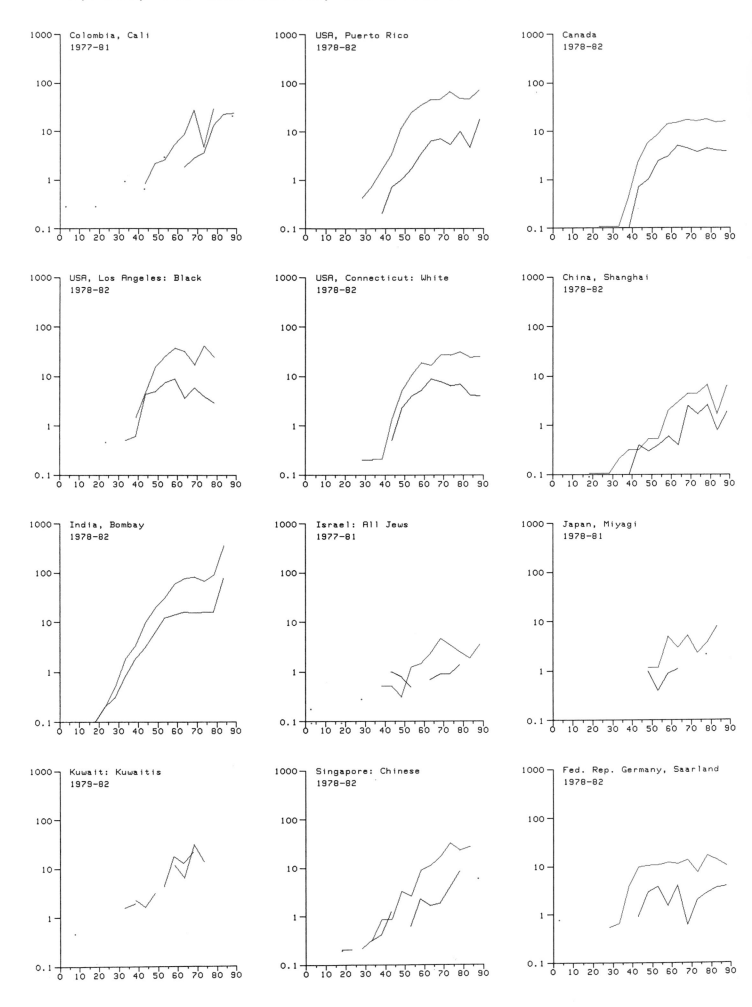

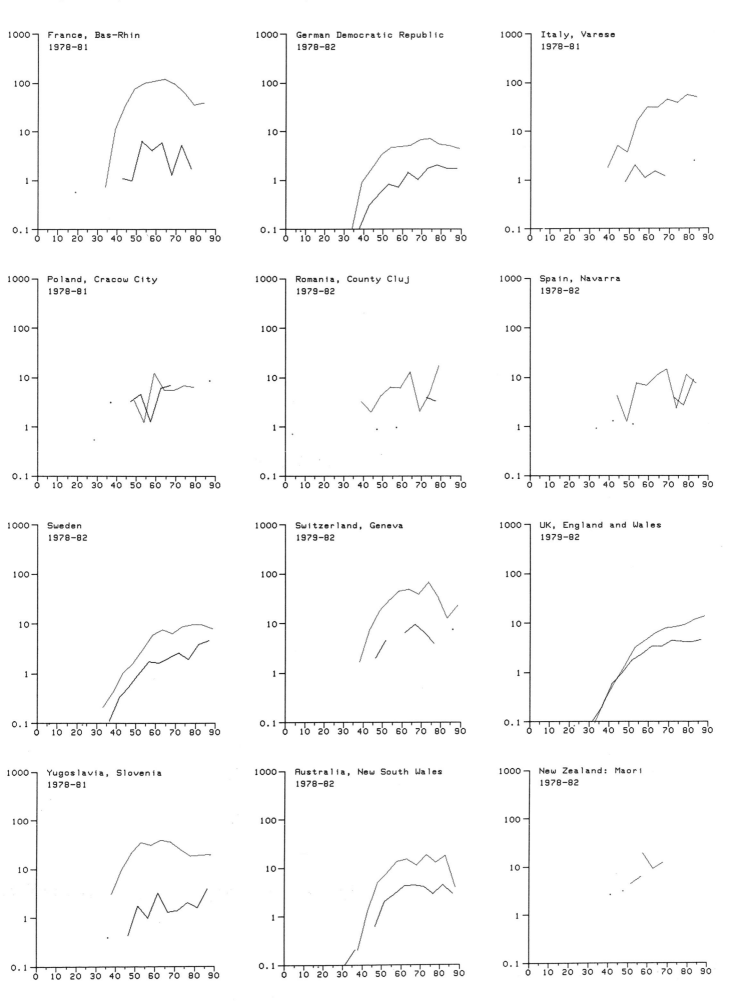

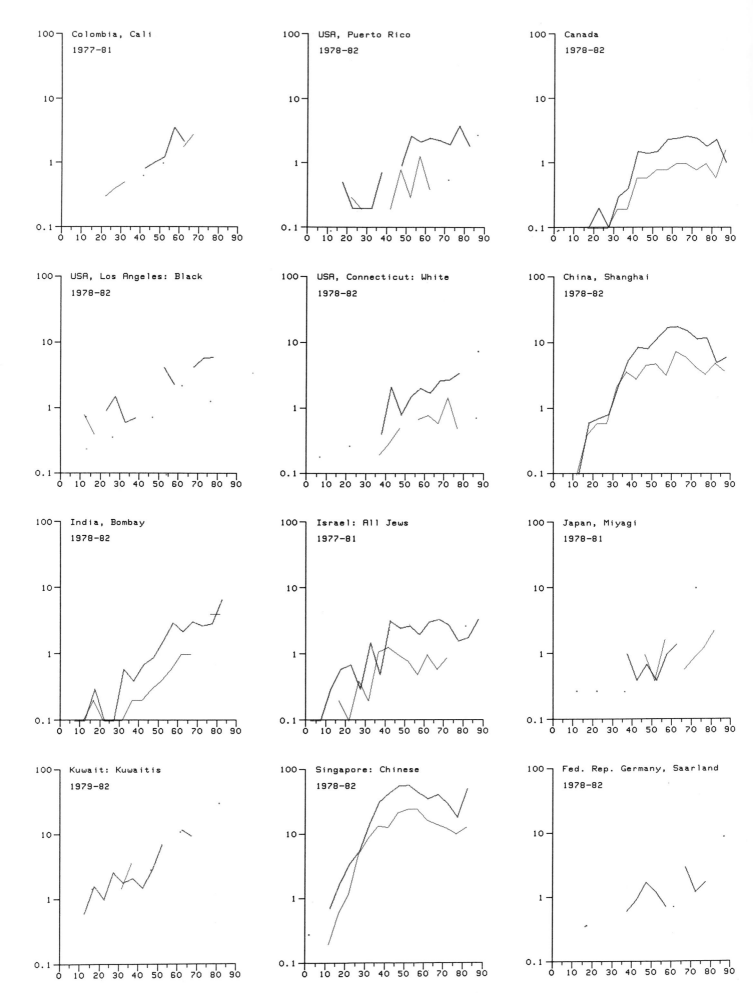

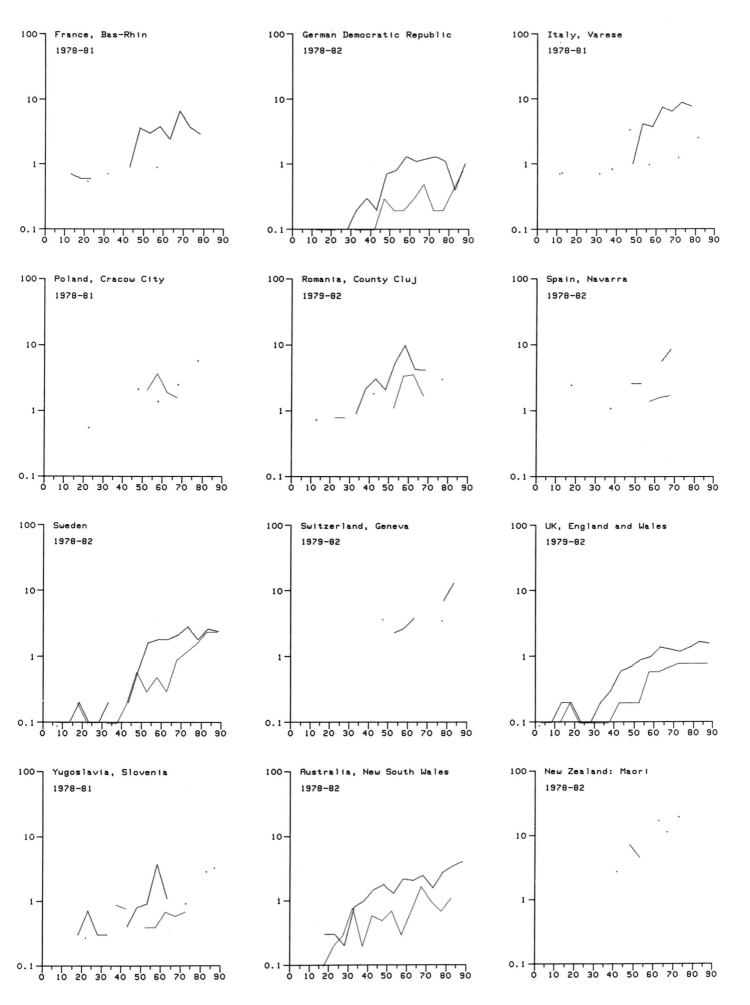

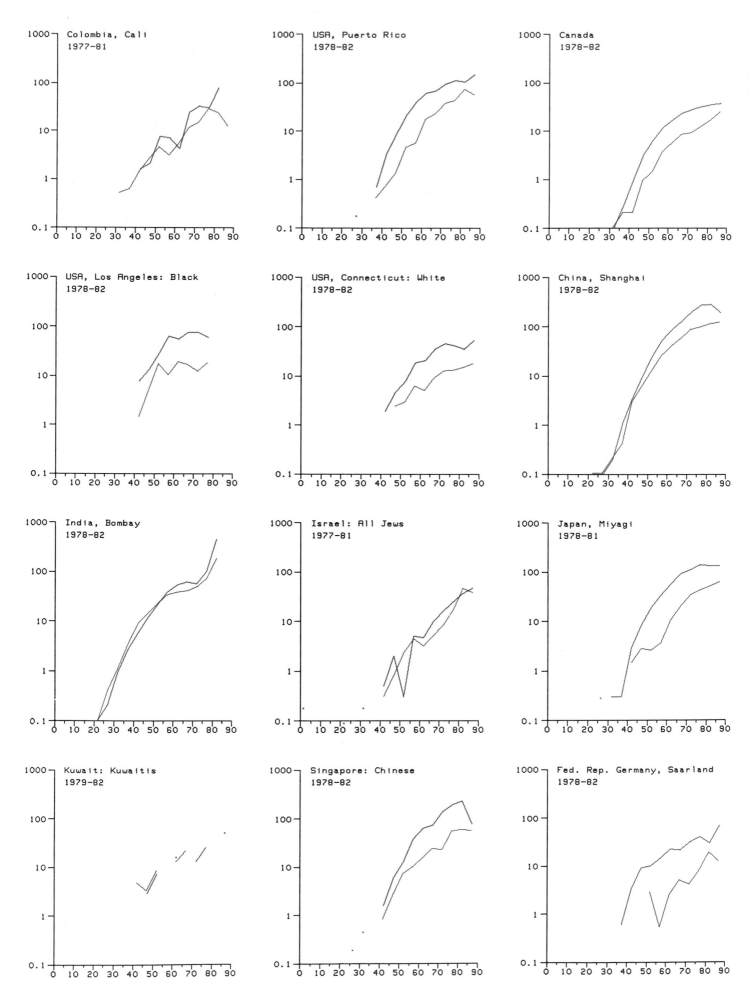

150 OESOPHAGUS

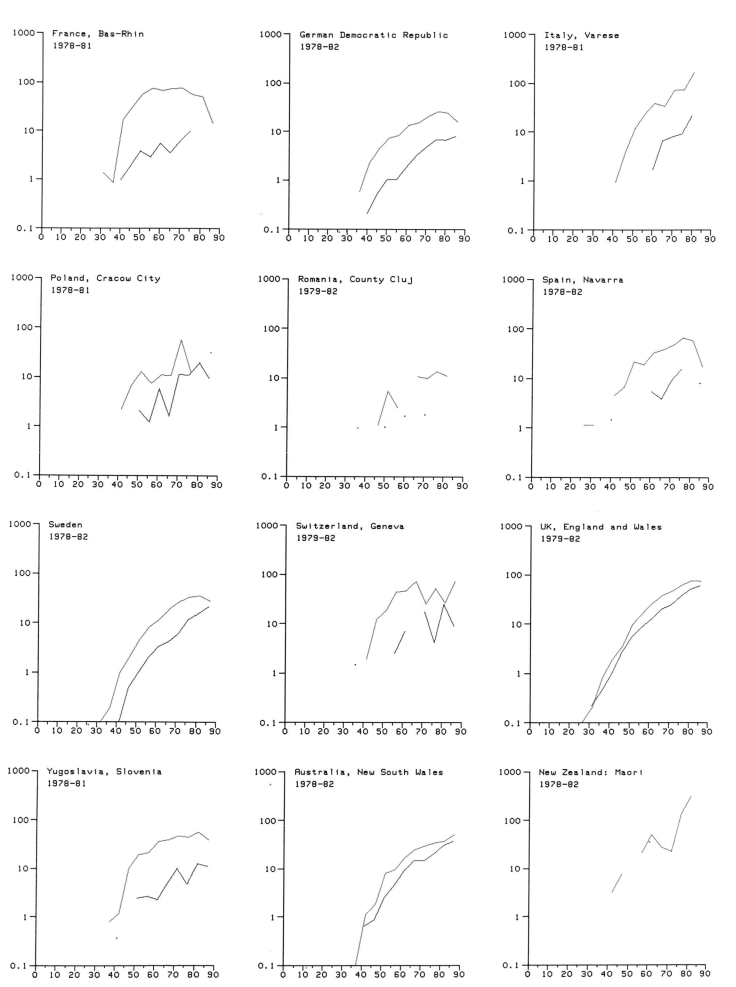

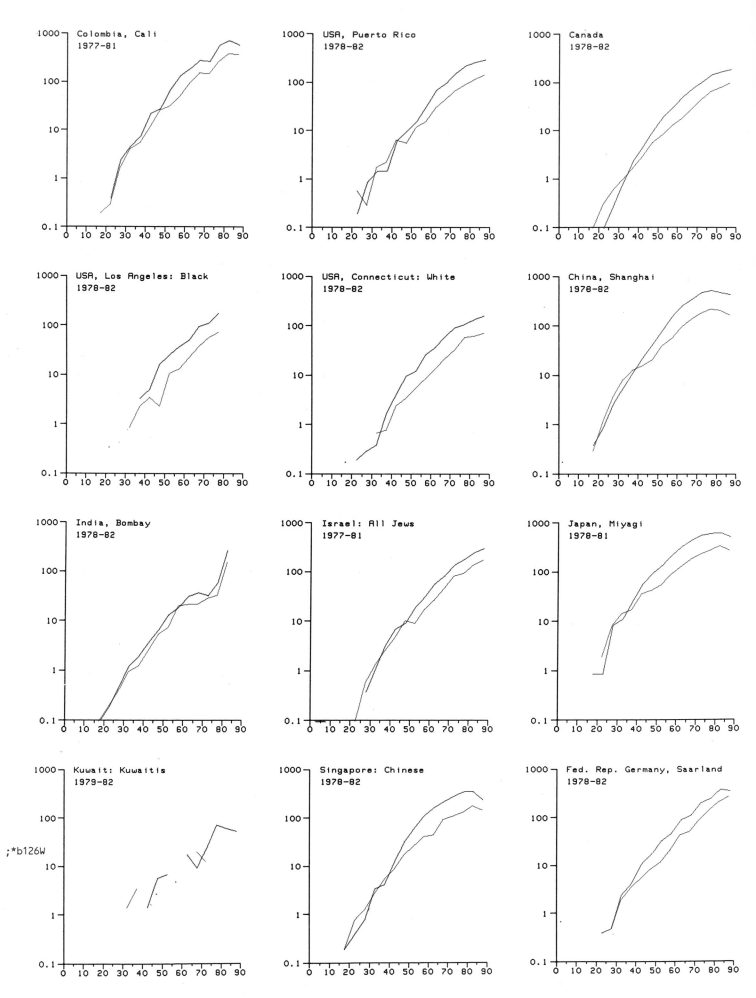

;*b126W

151 STOMACH

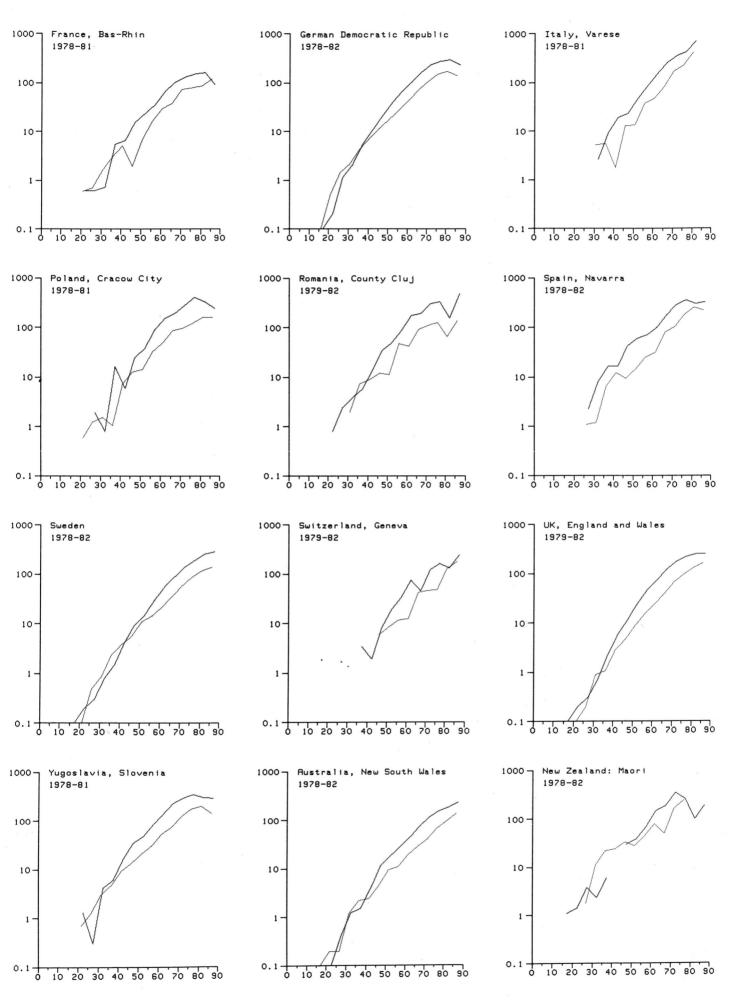

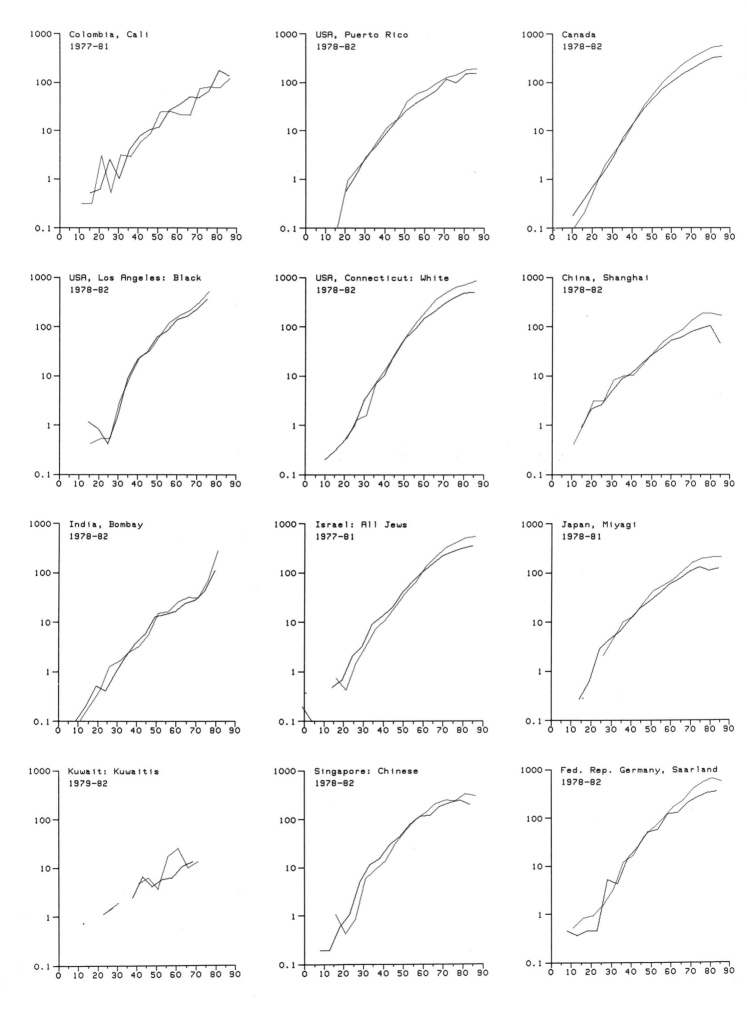

153-4 COLON + RECTUM

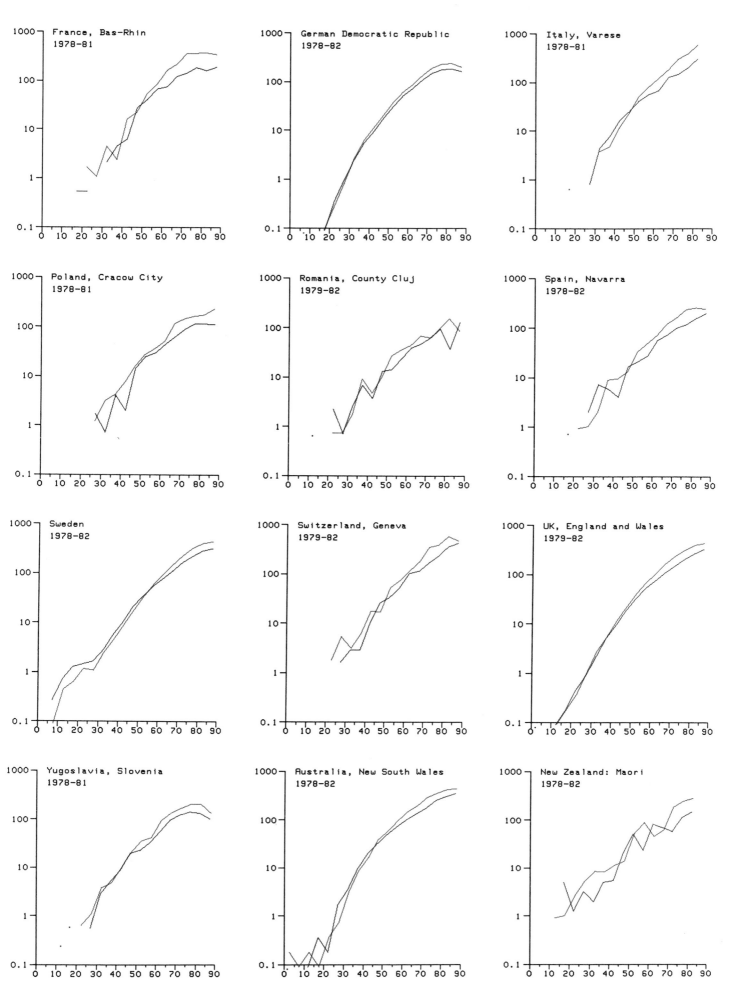

155 LIVER

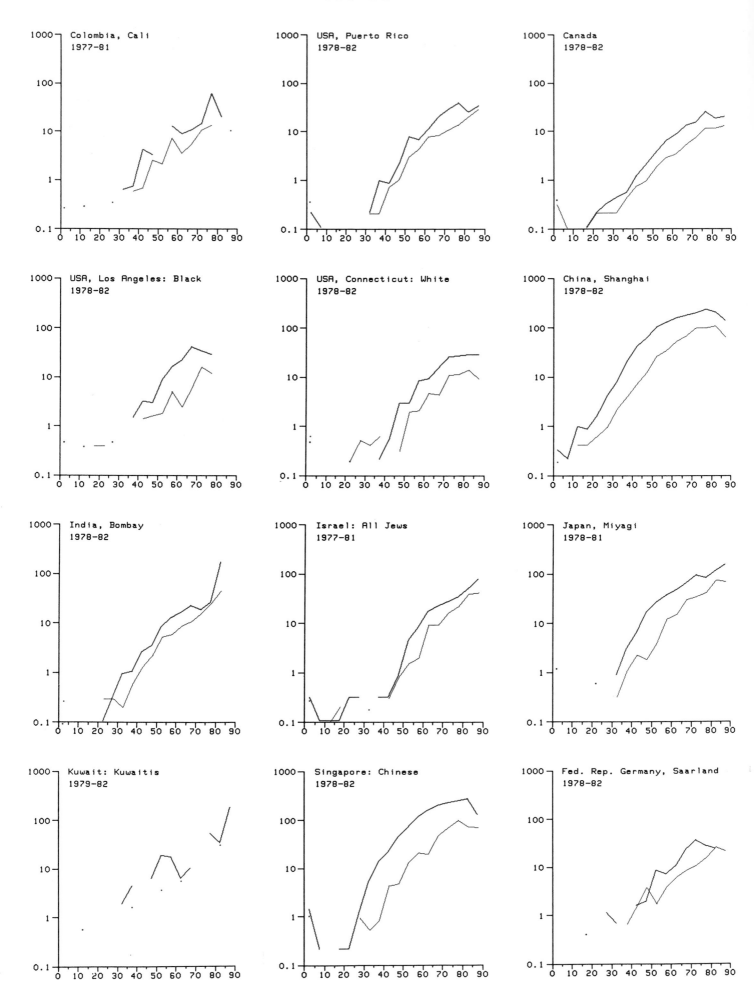

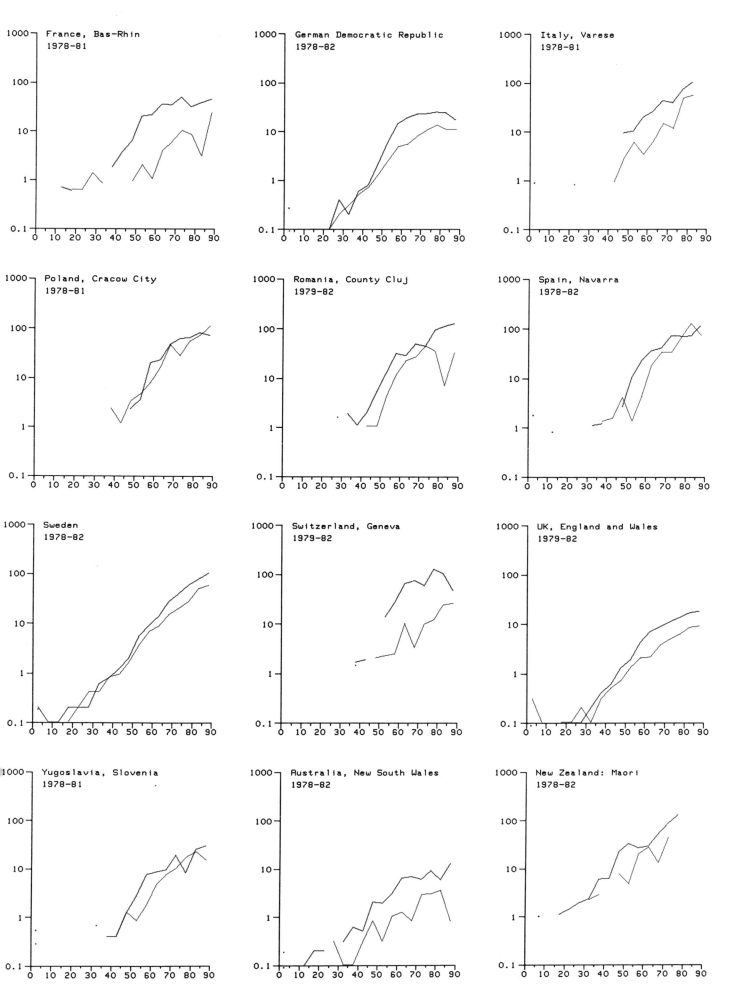

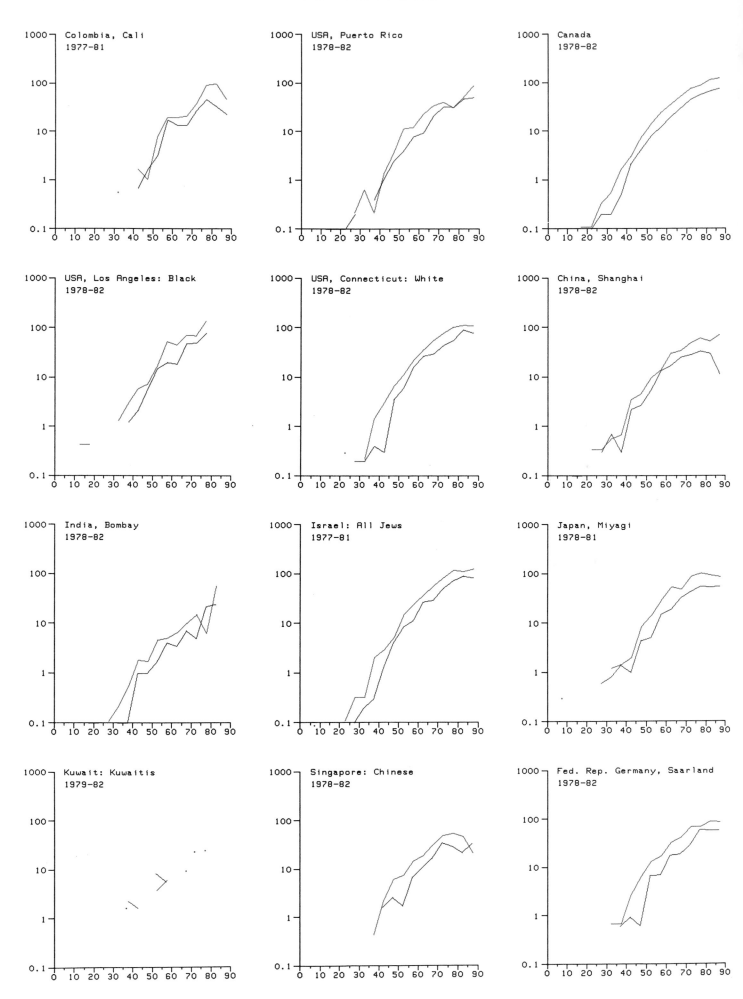

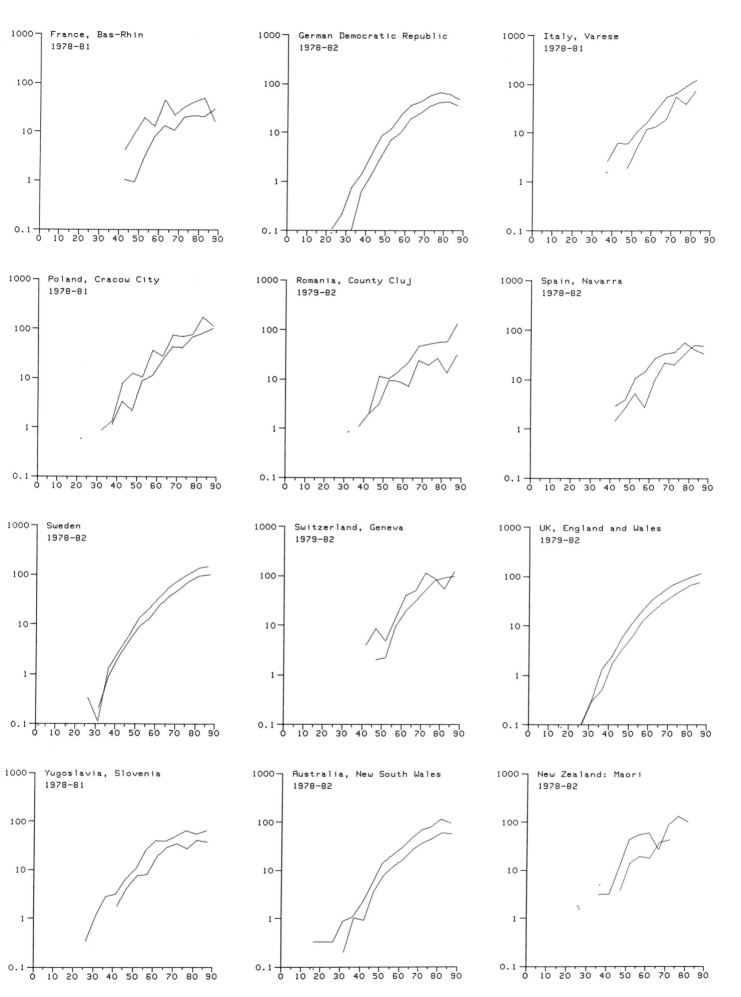

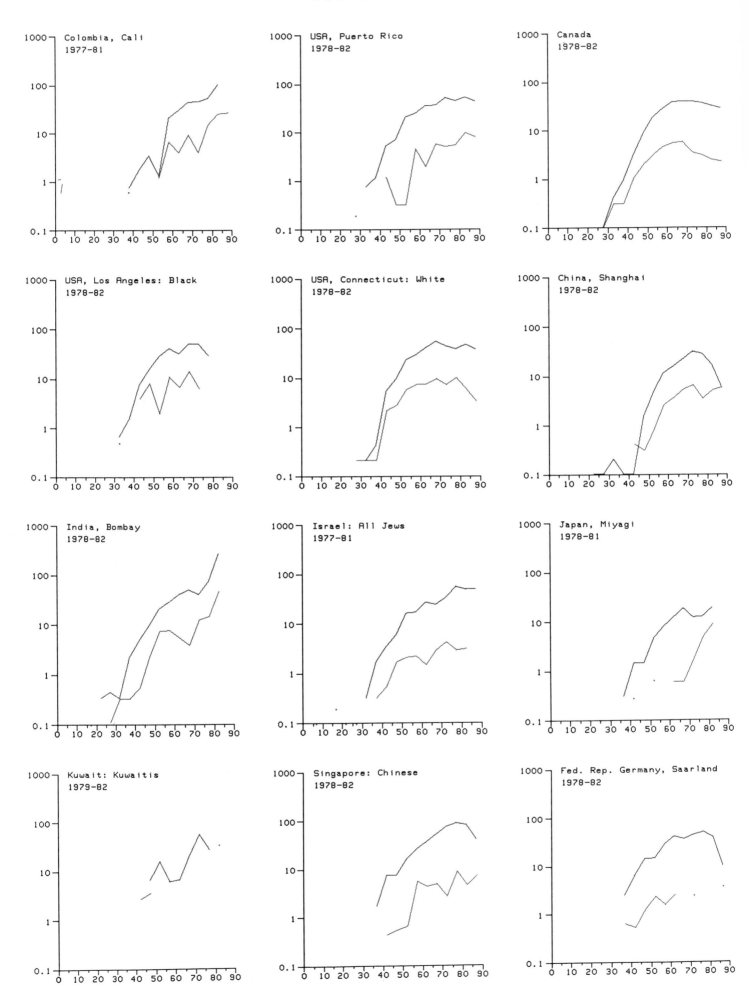

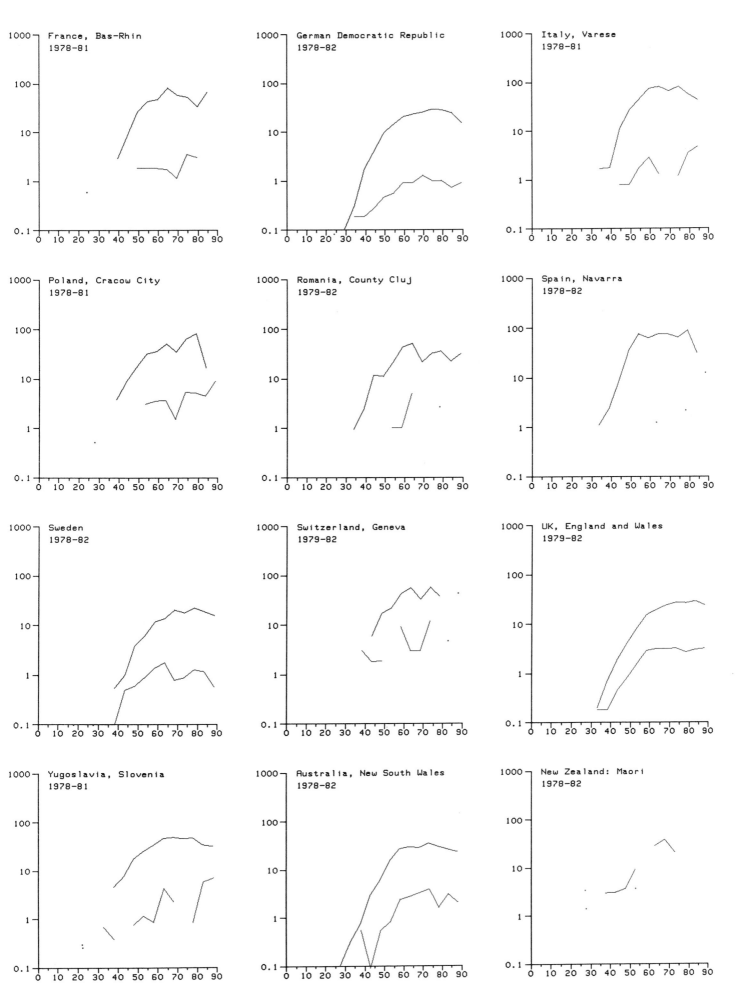

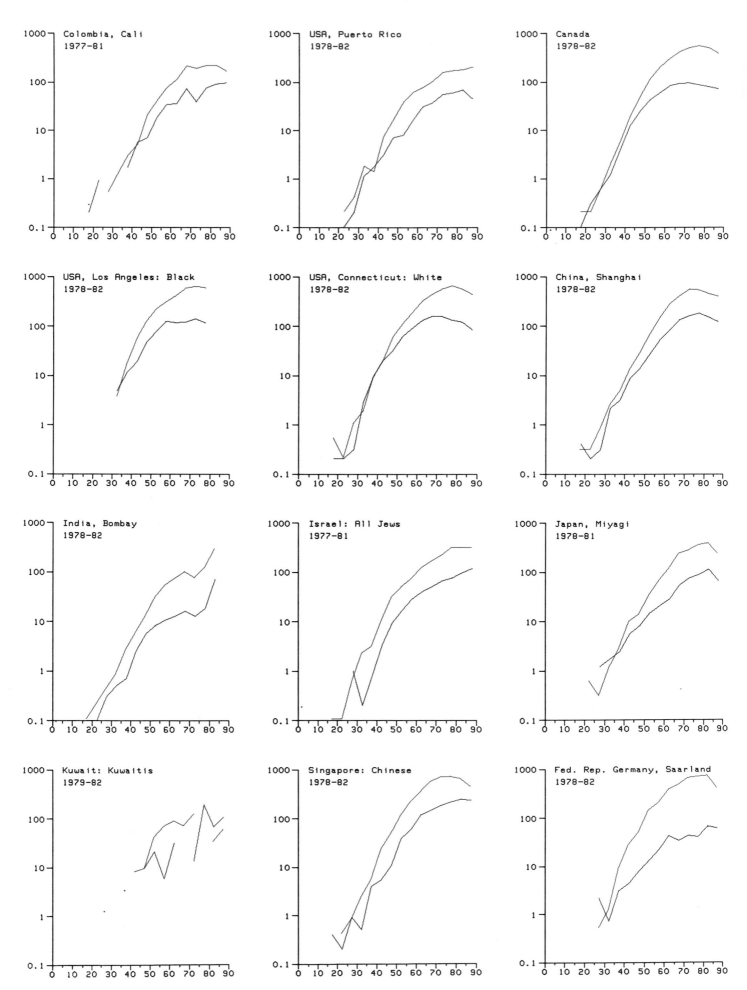

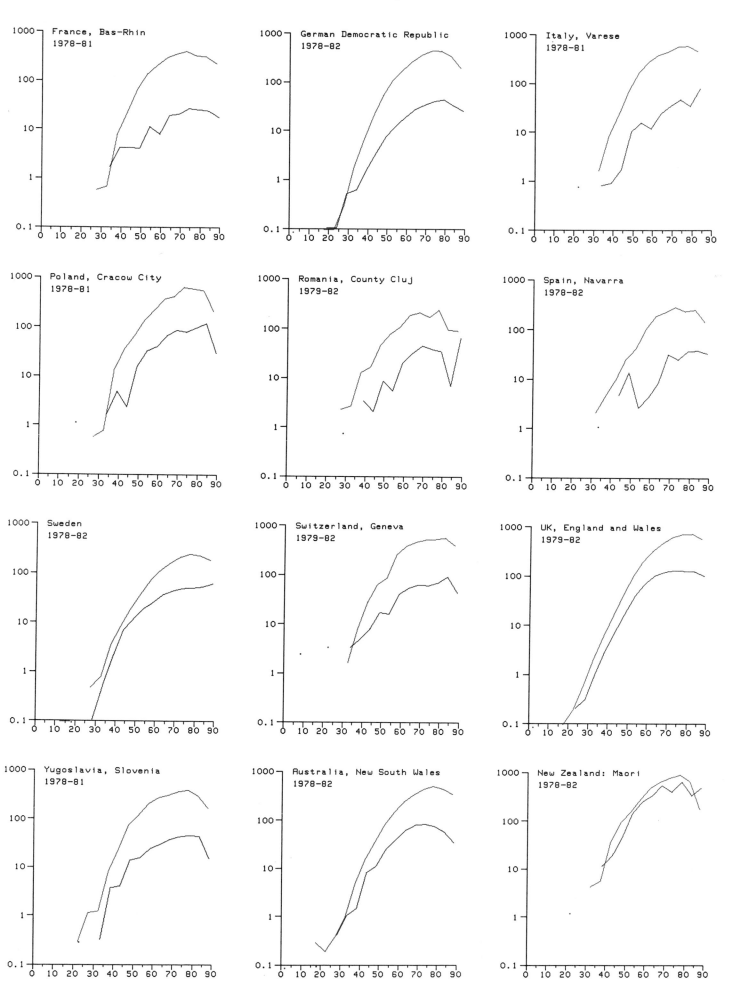

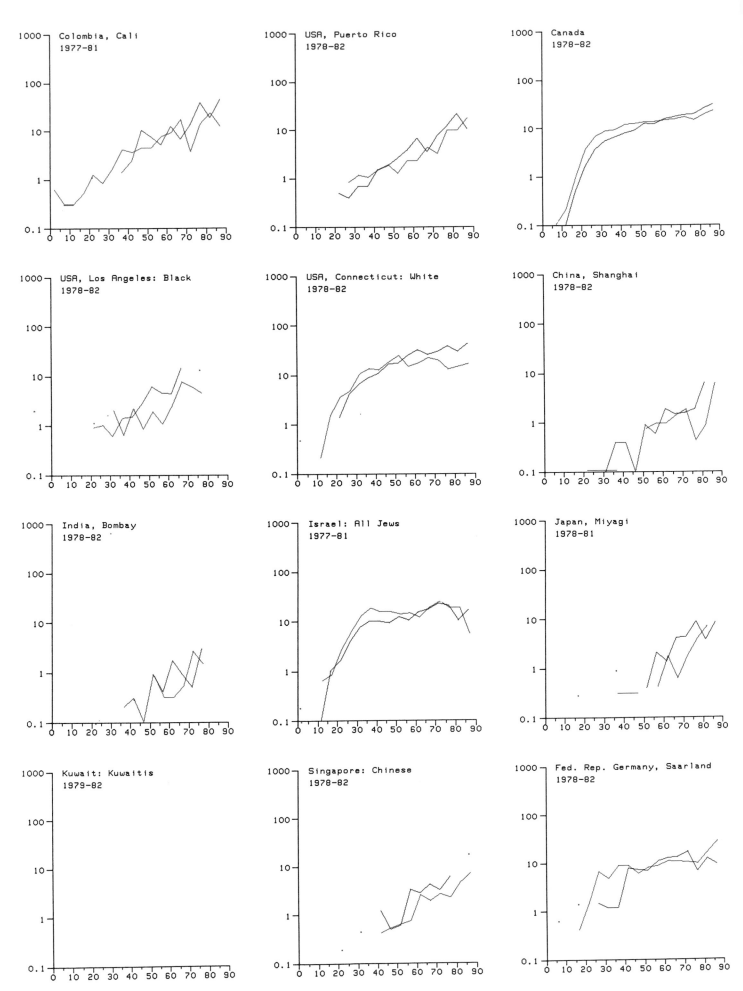

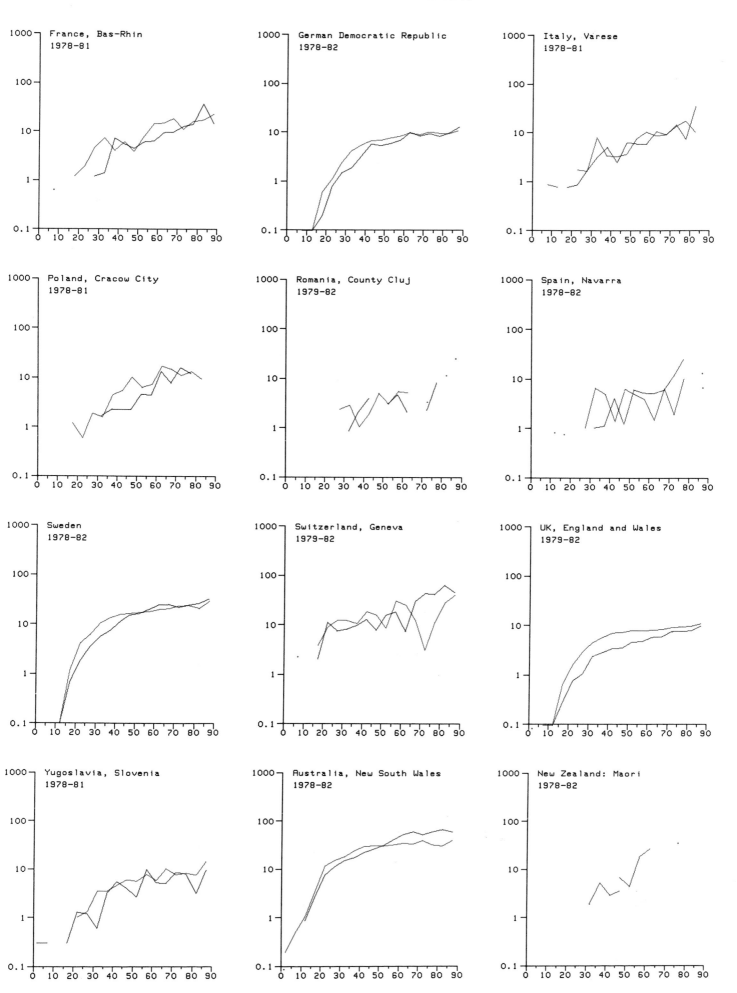

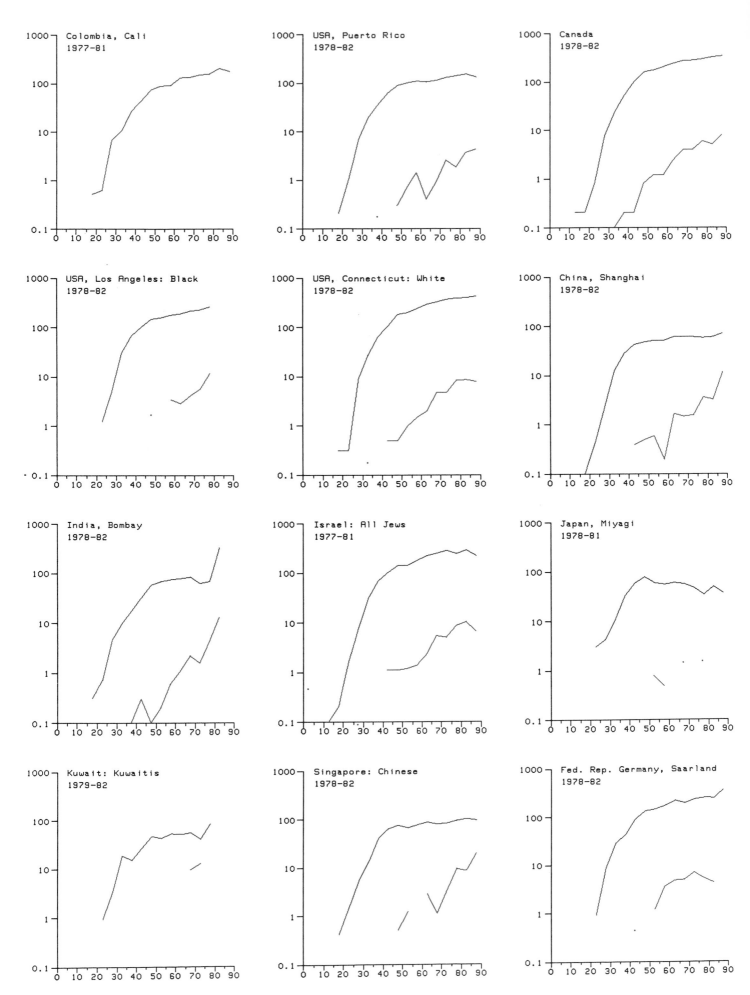

174-5 BREAST

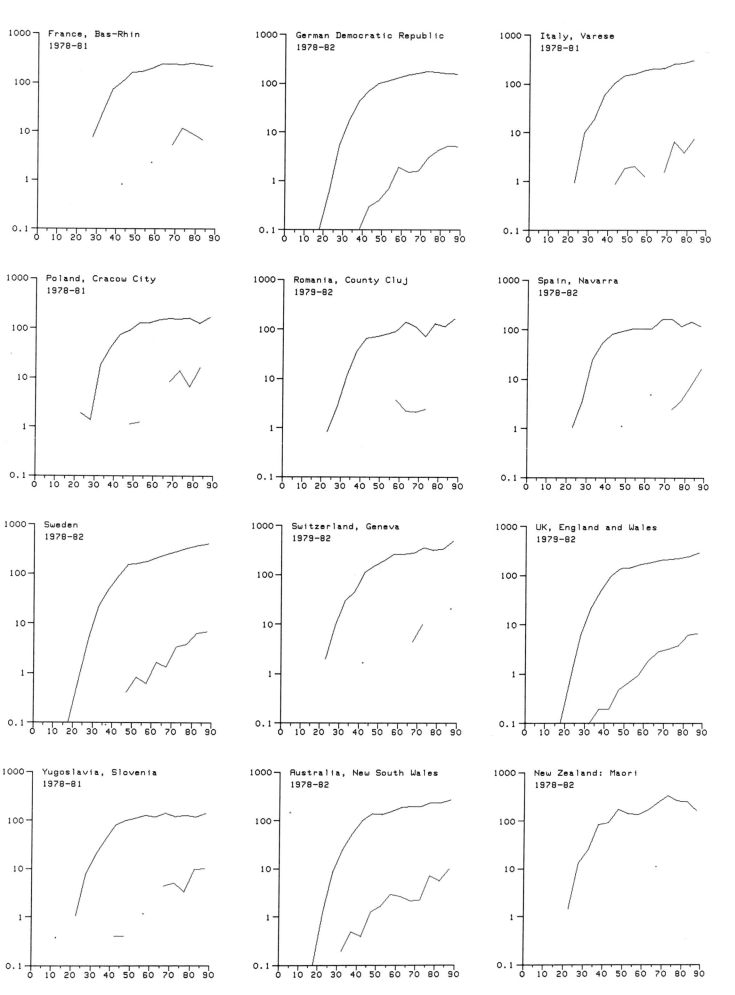

180 CERVIX UTERI

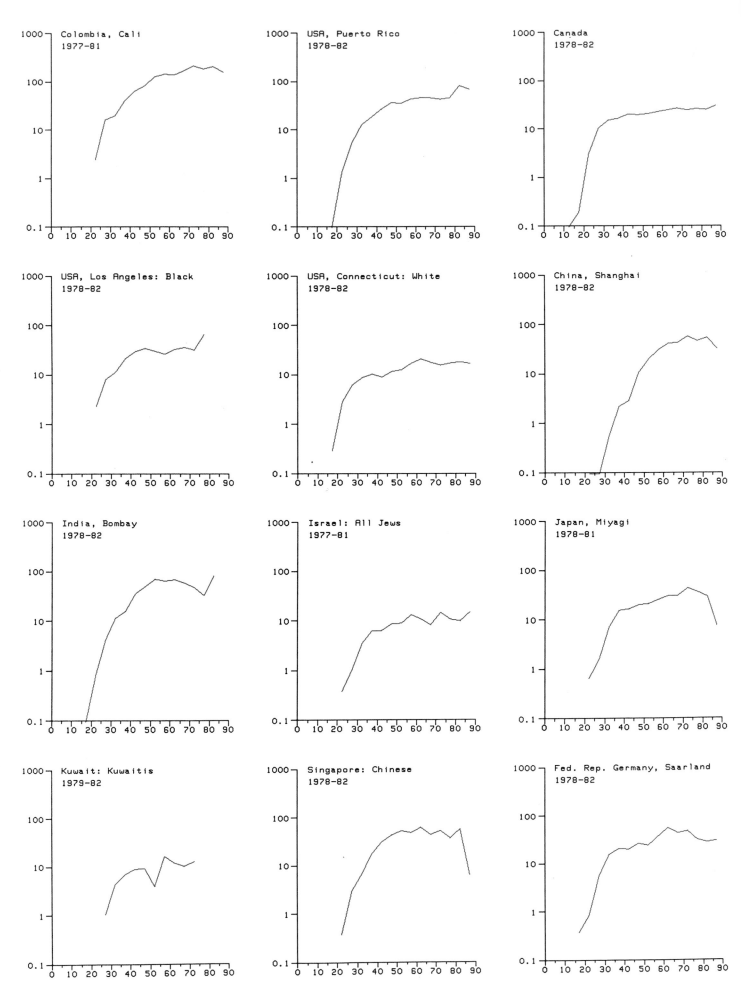

180 CERVIX UTERI

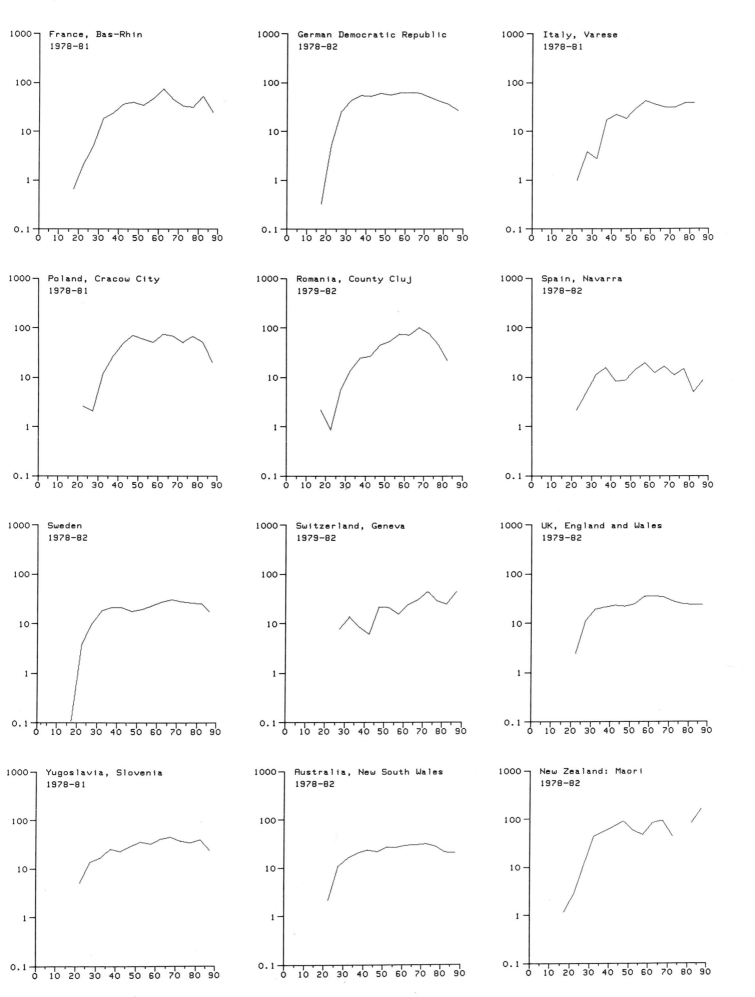

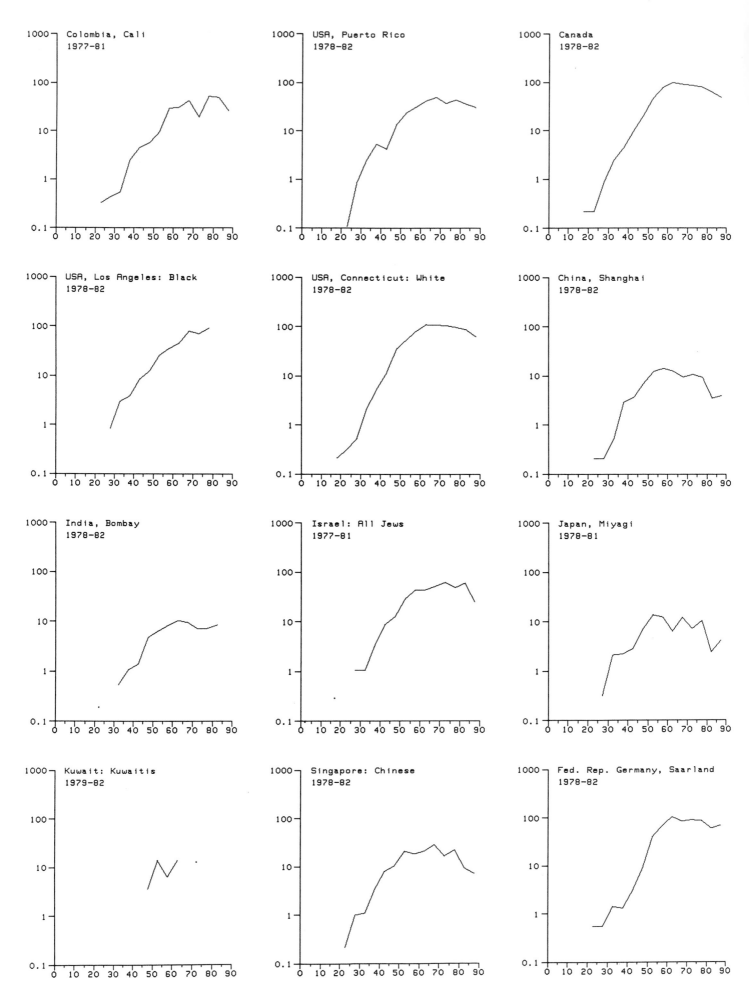

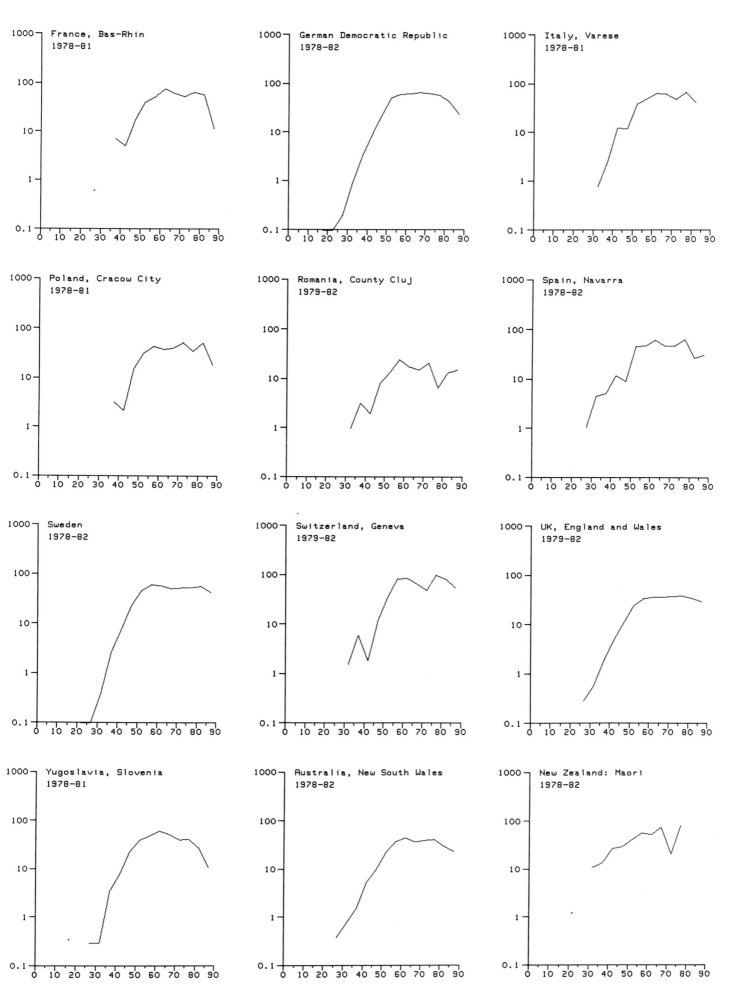

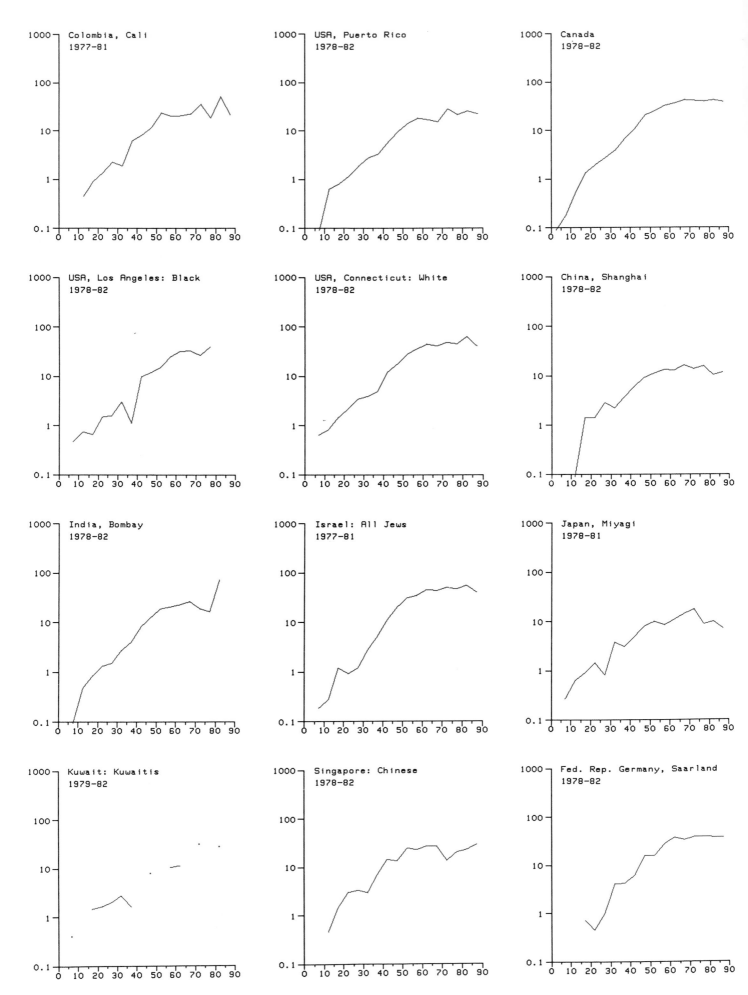

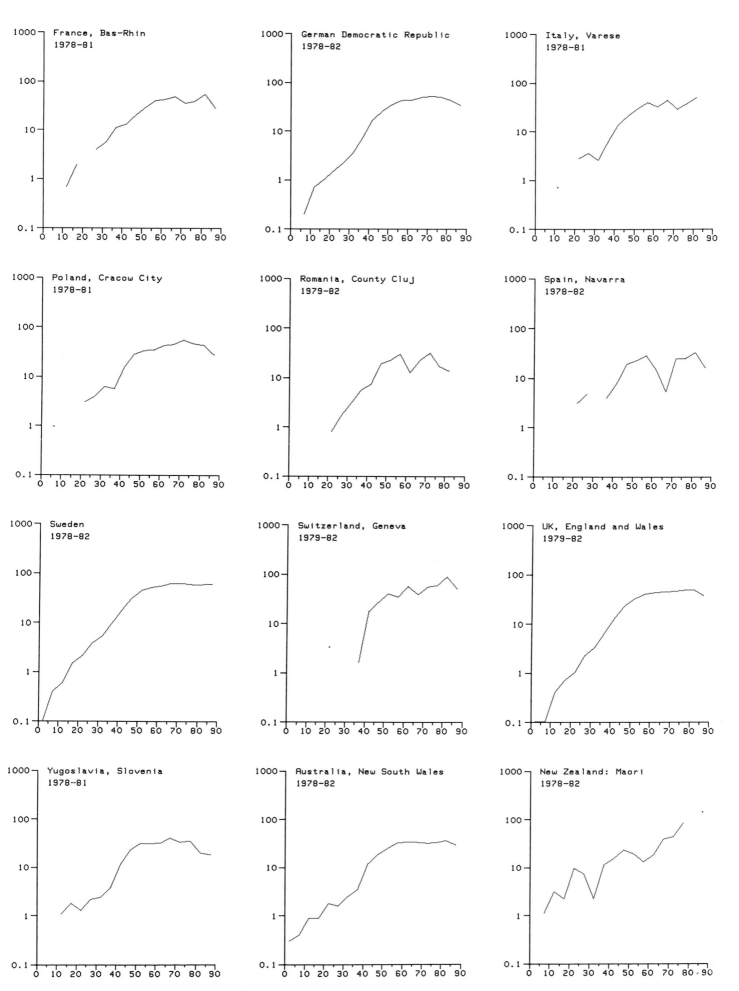

185 PROSTATE

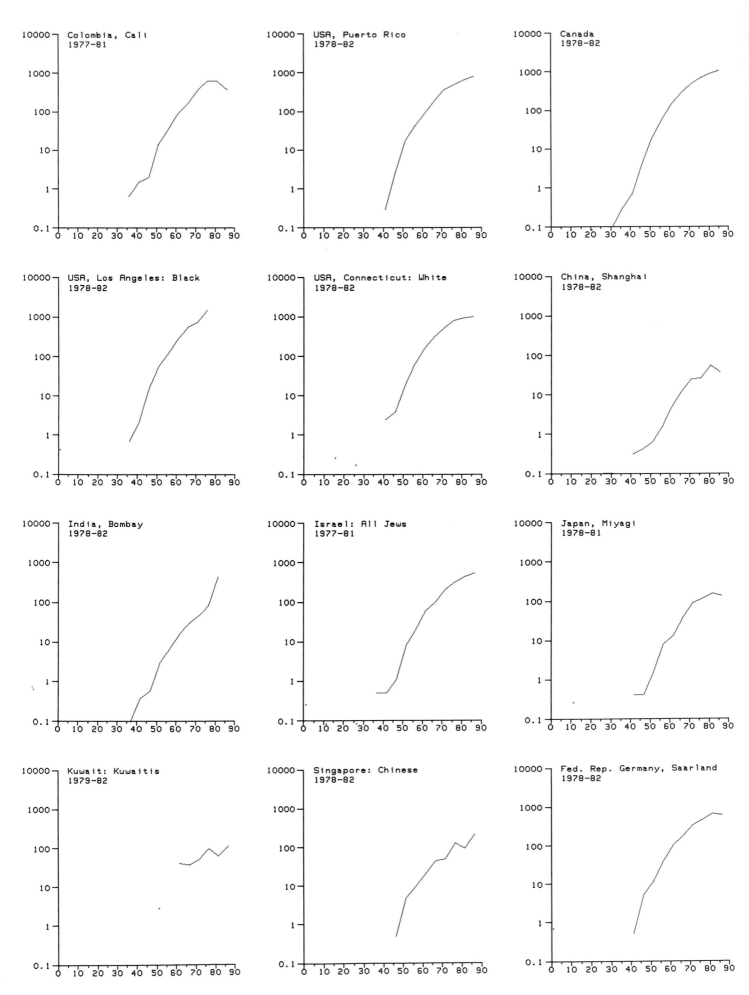

185 PROSTATE

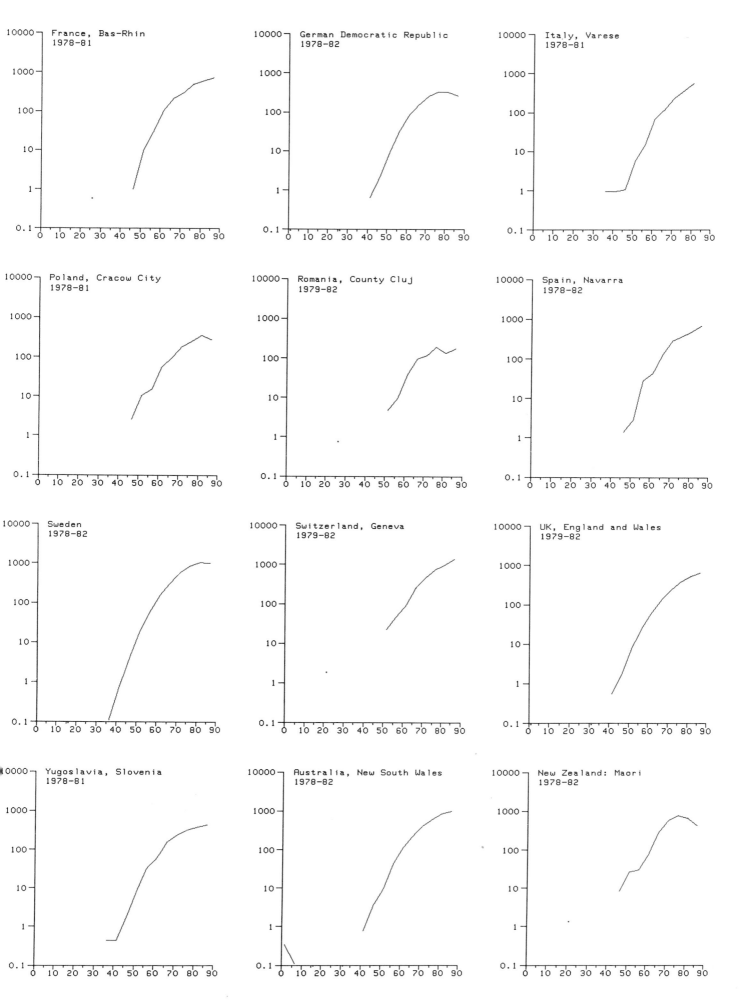

France, Bas-Rhin
1978-81

German Democratic Republic
1978-82

Italy, Varese
1978-81

Poland, Cracow City
1978-81

Romania, County Cluj
1979-82

Spain, Navarra
1978-82

Sweden
1978-82

Switzerland, Geneva
1979-82

UK, England and Wales
1979-82

Yugoslavia, Slovenia
1978-81

Australia, New South Wales
1978-82

New Zealand: Maori
1978-82

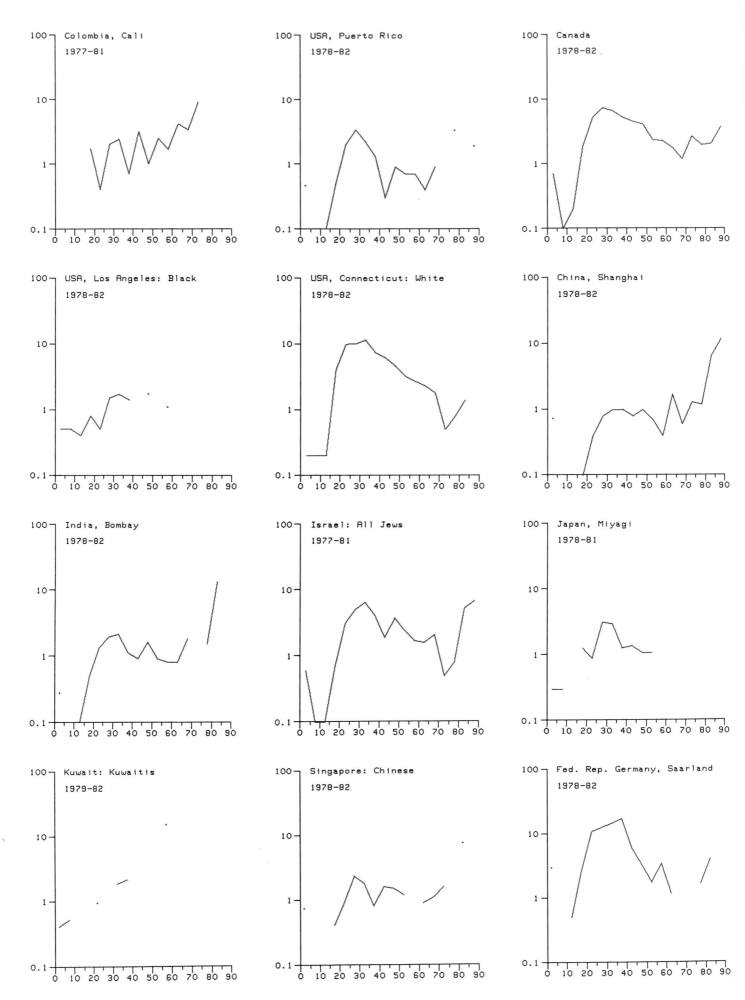

186 TESTIS

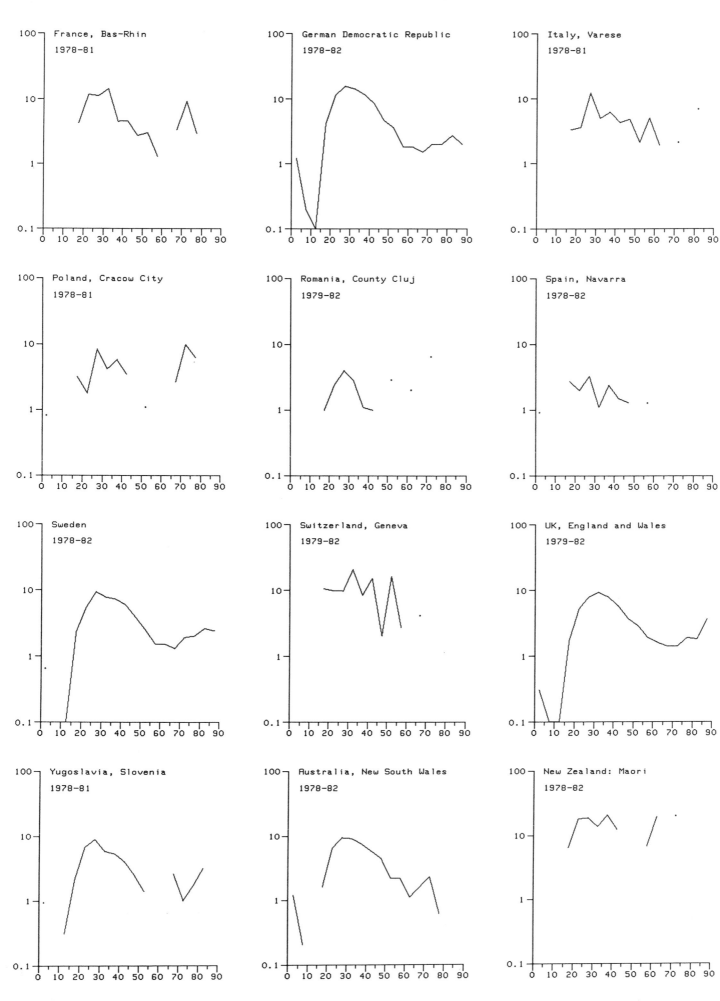

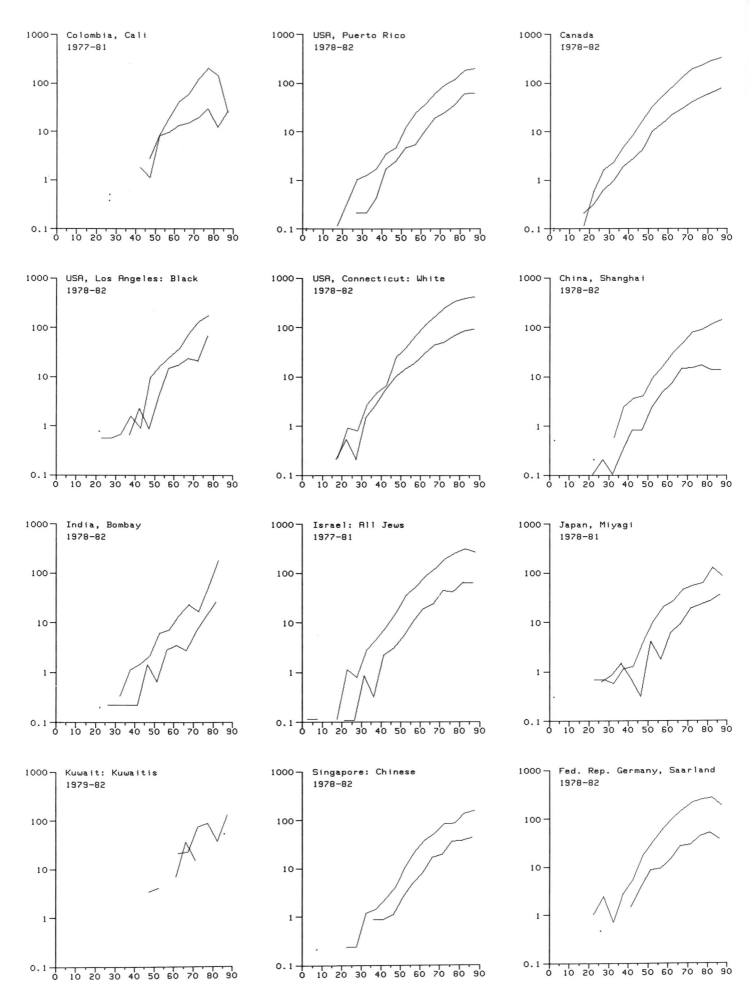

188 BLADDER

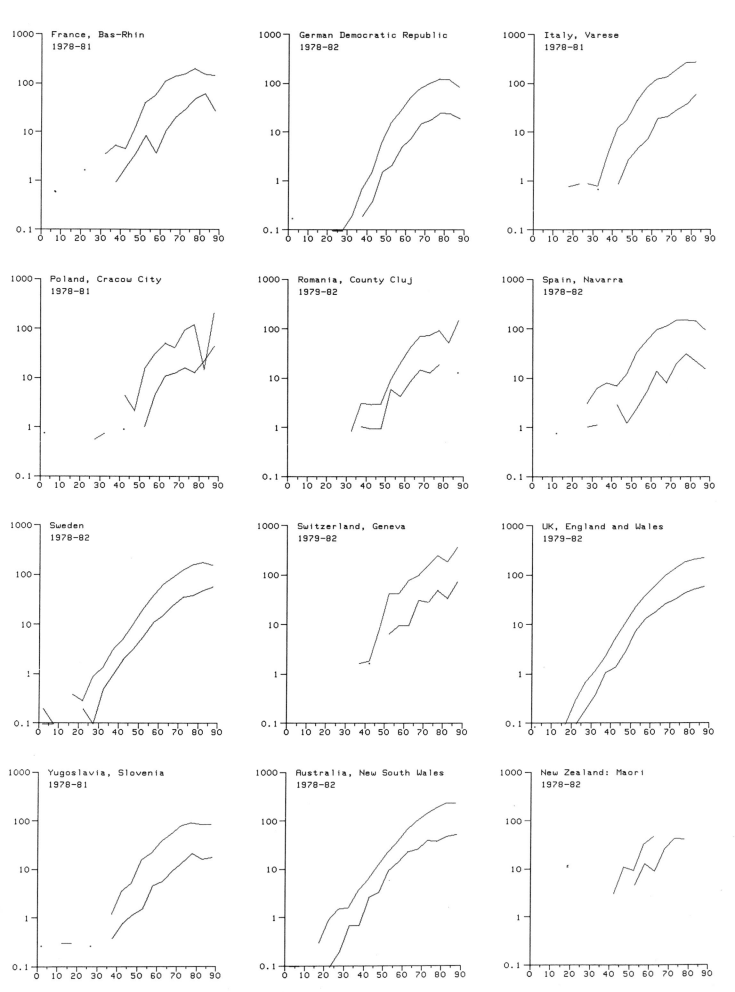

189 OTHER URINARY

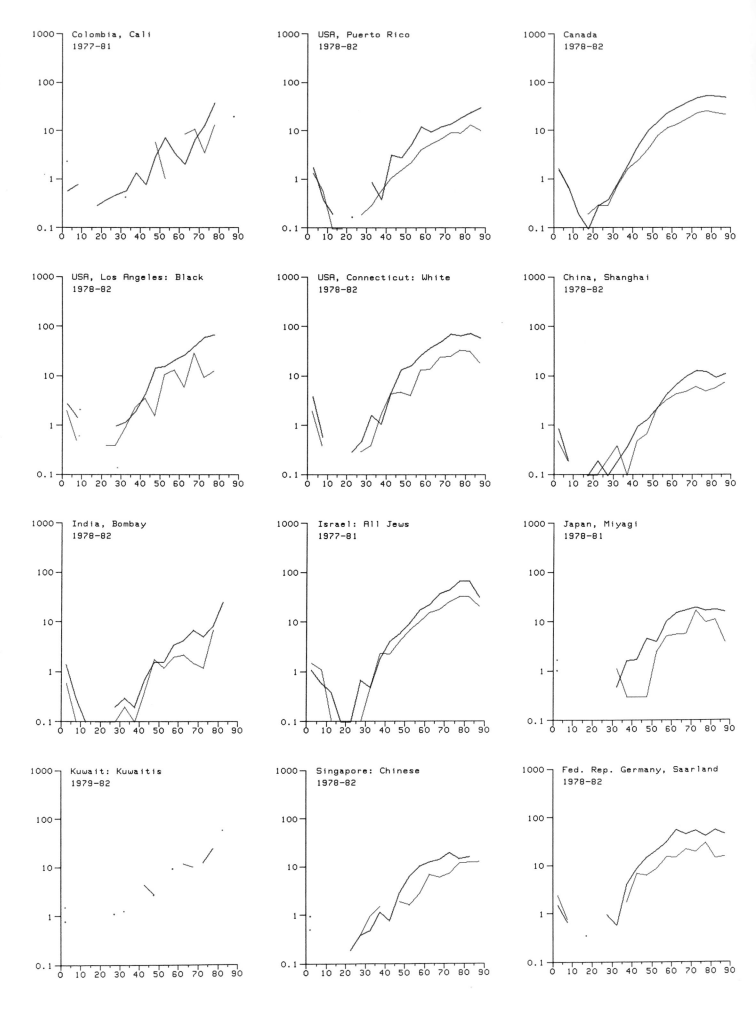

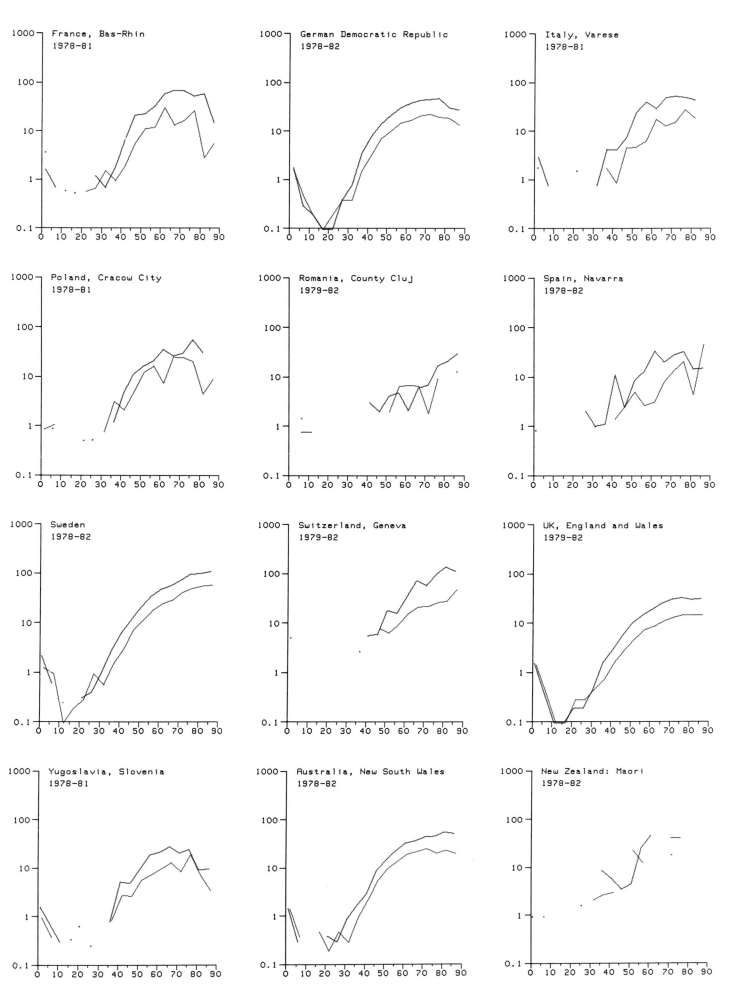

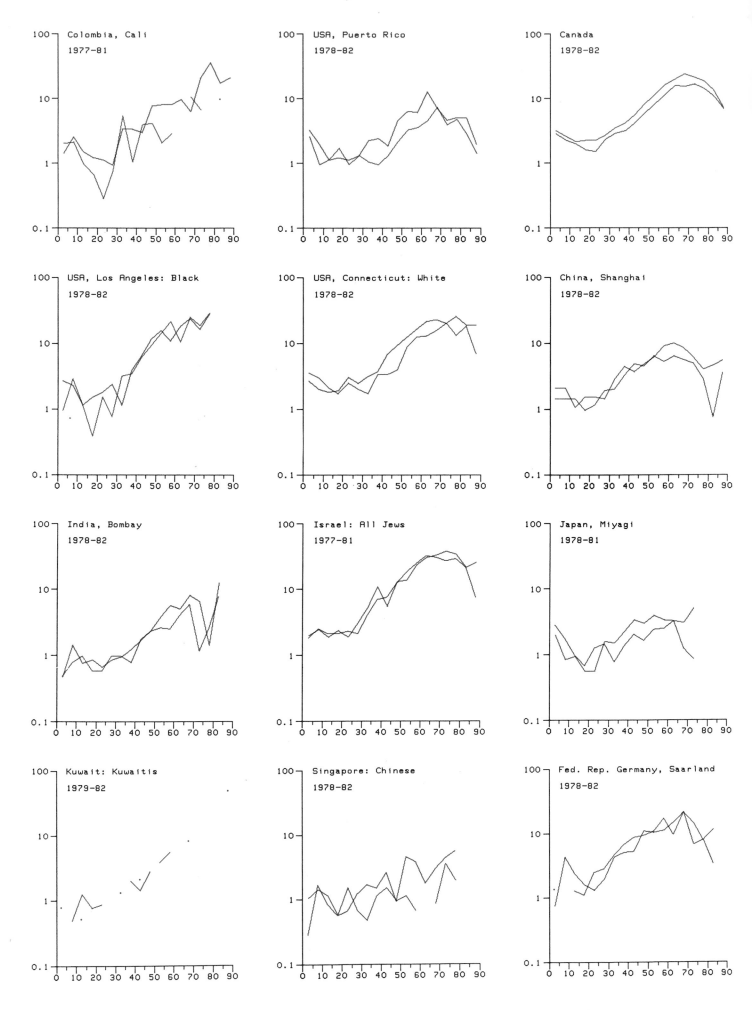

191-2 BRAIN, NERVOUS SYSTEM

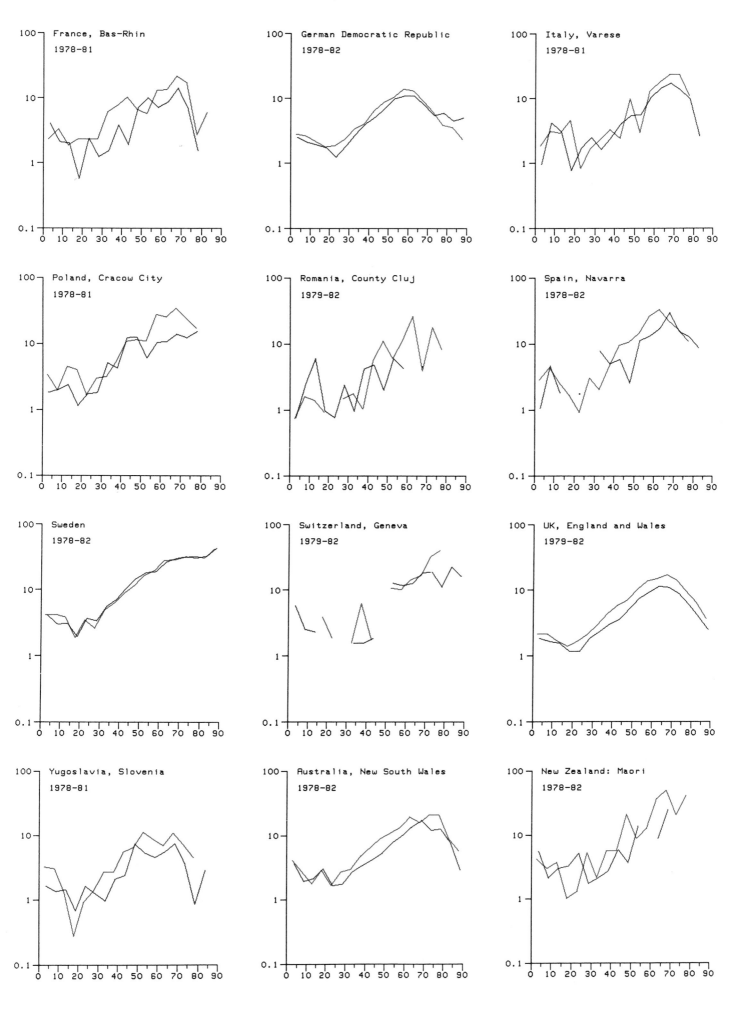

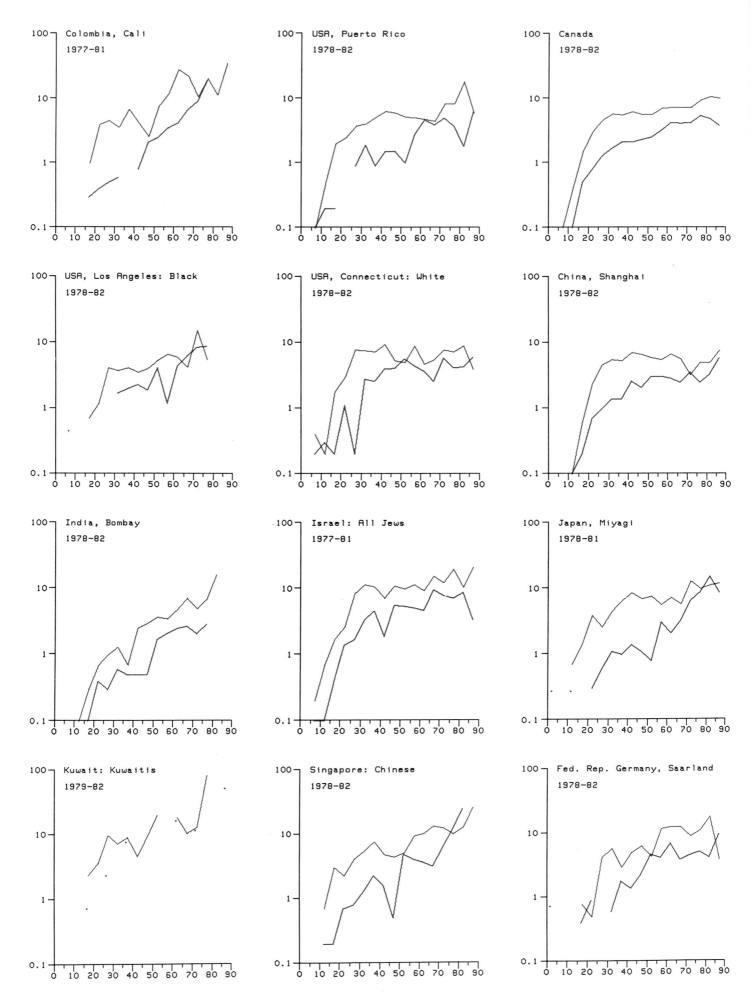

193 THYROID

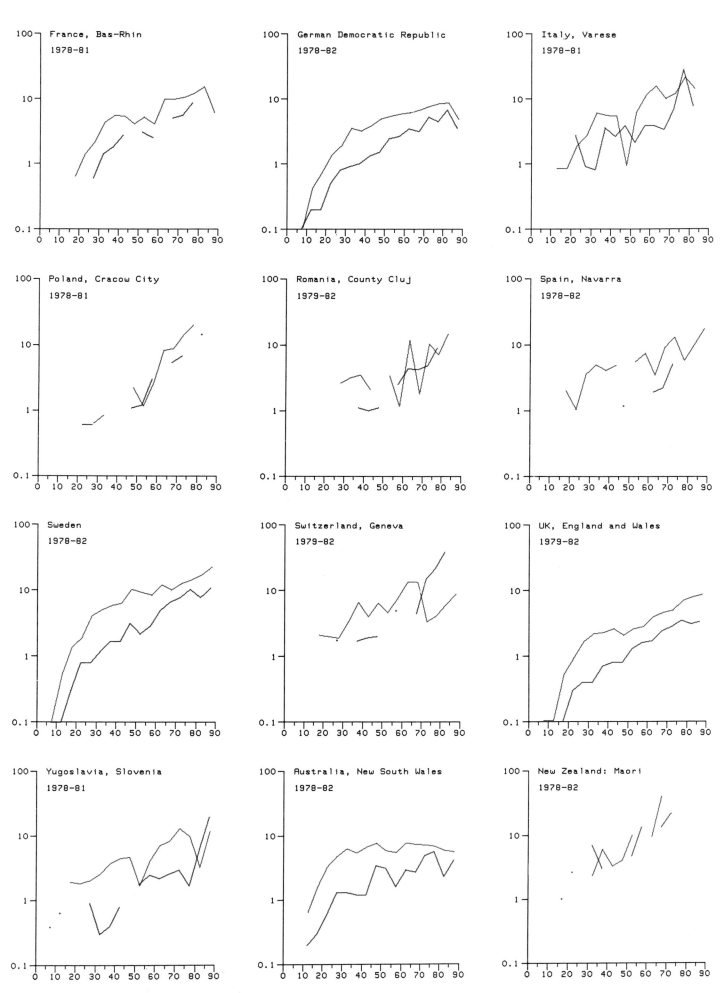

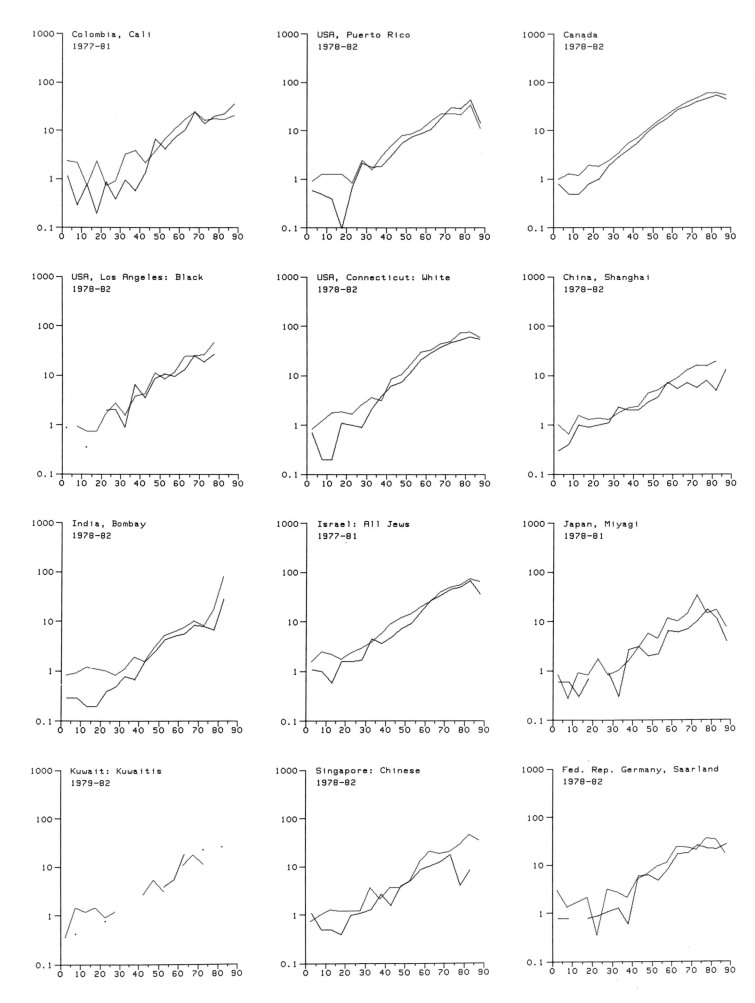

200 + 202 NON-HODGKIN LYMPHOMA

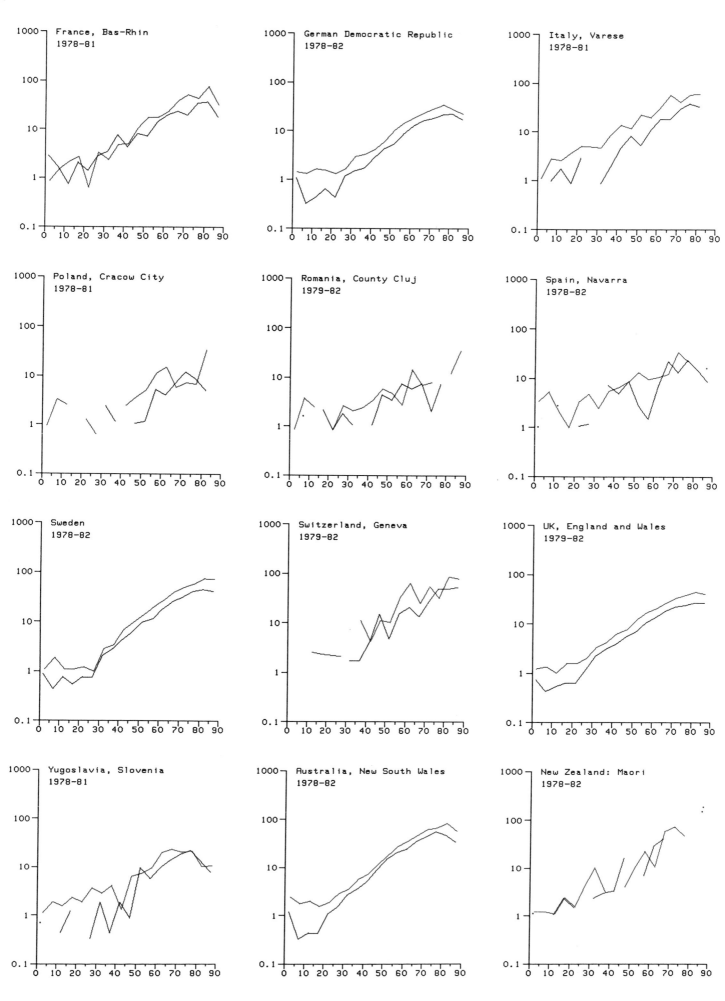

201 HODGKIN'S DISEASE

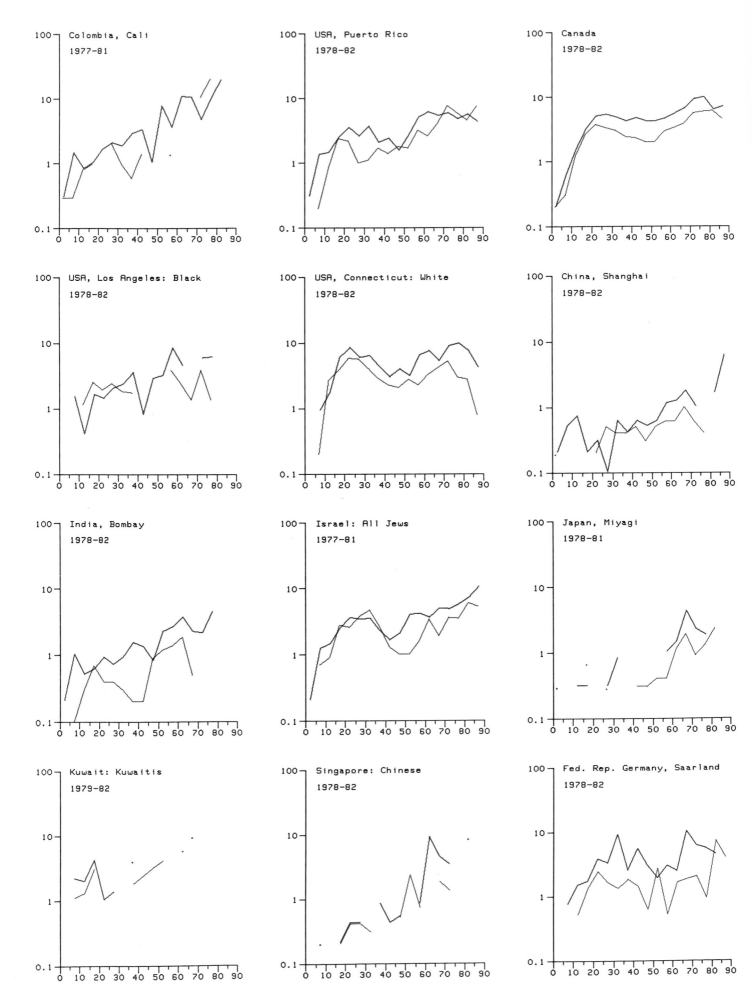

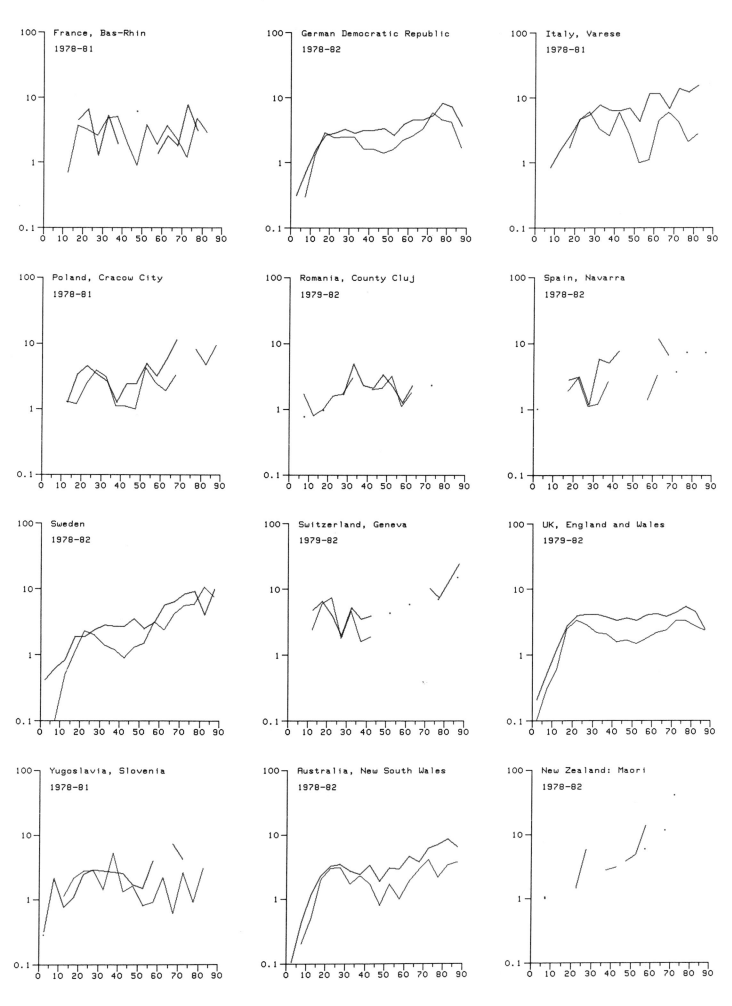

204-8 LEUKAEMIA

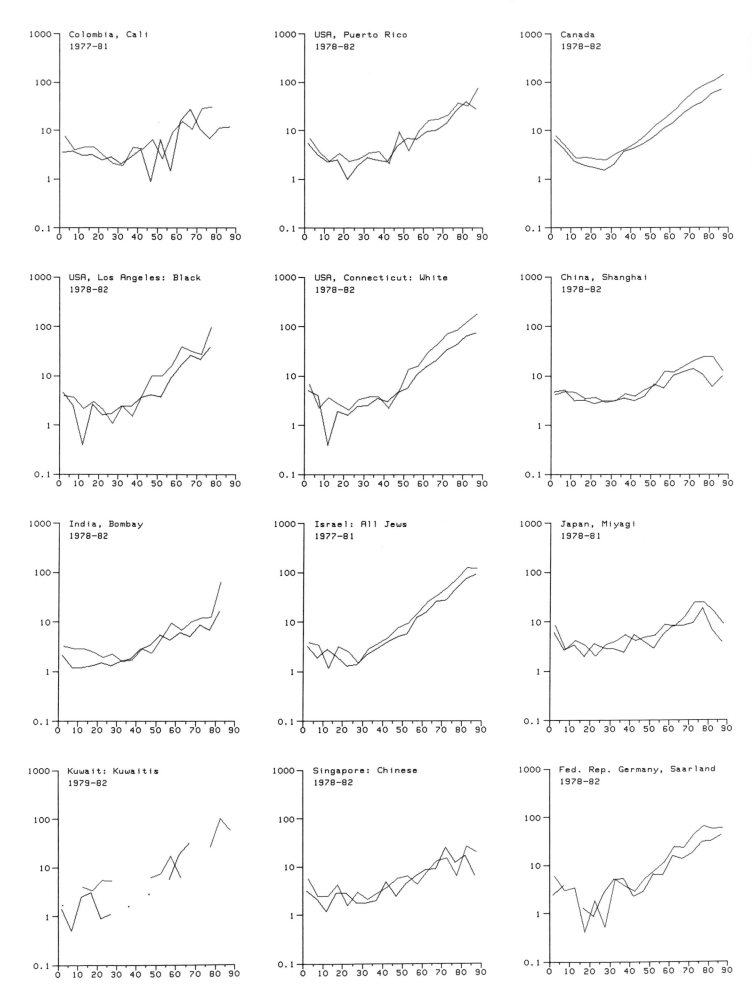

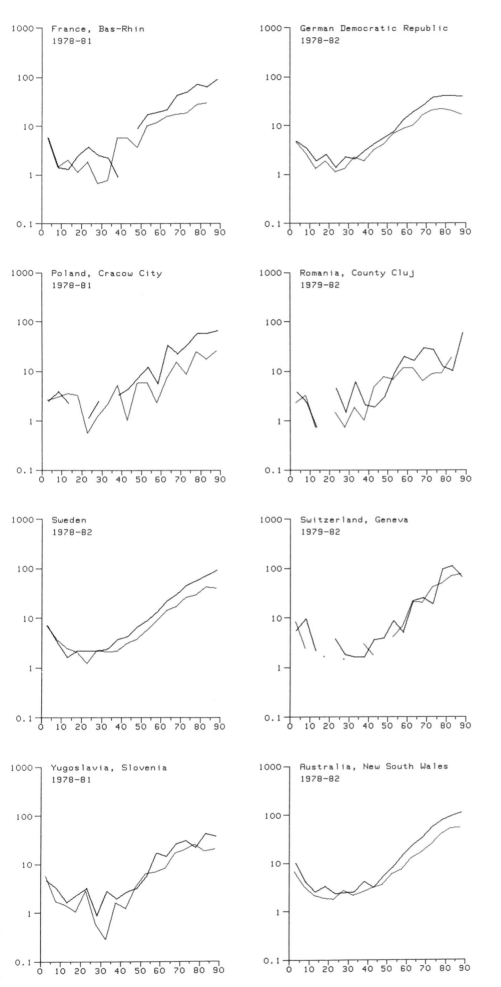

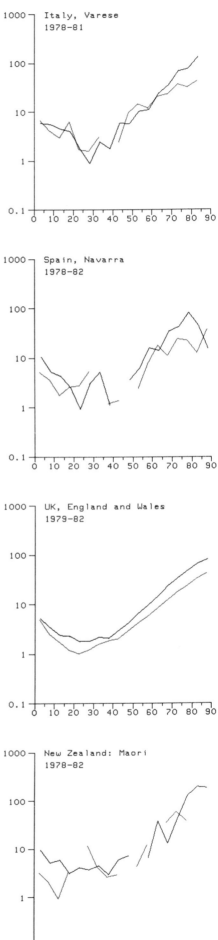

PUBLICATIONS OF THE INTERNATIONAL
AGENCY FOR RESEARCH ON CANCER
Scientific Publications Series

(Available from Oxford University Press through local bookshops)

No. 1 Liver Cancer
1971; 176 pages (*out of print*)

No. 2 Oncogenesis and Herpesviruses
Edited by P.M. Biggs, G. de-Thé and L.N. Payne
1972; 515 pages (*out of print*)

No. 3 N-Nitroso Compounds: Analysis and Formation
Edited by P. Bogovski, R. Preussman and E.A. Walker
1972; 140 pages (*out of print*)

No. 4 Transplacental Carcinogenesis
Edited by L. Tomatis and U. Mohr
1973; 181 pages (*out of print*)

No. 5/6 Pathology of Tumours in Laboratory Animals, Volume 1, Tumours of the Rat
Edited by V.S. Turusov
1973/1976; 533 pages; £50.00

No. 7 Host Environment Interactions in the Etiology of Cancer in Man
Edited by R. Doll and I. Vodopija
1973; 464 pages; £32.50

No. 8 Biological Effects of Asbestos
Edited by P. Bogovski, J.C. Gilson, V. Timbrell and J.C. Wagner
1973; 346 pages (*out of print*)

No. 9 N-Nitroso Compounds in the Environment
Edited by P. Bogovski and E.A. Walker
1974; 243 pages; £21.00

No. 10 Chemical Carcinogenesis Essays
Edited by R. Montesano and L. Tomatis
1974; 230 pages (*out of print*)

No. 11 Oncogenesis and Herpesviruses II
Edited by G. de-Thé, M.A. Epstein and H. zur Hausen
1975; Part I: 511 pages
Part II: 403 pages; £65.00

No. 12 Screening Tests in Chemical Carcinogenesis
Edited by R. Montesano, H. Bartsch and L. Tomatis
1976; 666 pages; £45.00

No. 13 Environmental Pollution and Carcinogenic Risks
Edited by C. Rosenfeld and W. Davis
1975; 441 pages (*out of print*)

No. 14 Environmental N-Nitroso Compounds. Analysis and Formation
Edited by E.A. Walker, P. Bogovski and L. Griciute
1976; 512 pages; £37.50

No. 15 Cancer Incidence in Five Continents, Volume III
Edited by J.A.H. Waterhouse, C. Muir, P. Correa and J. Powell
1976; 584 pages; (*out of print*)

No. 16 Air Pollution and Cancer in Man
Edited by U. Mohr, D. Schmähl and L. Tomatis
1977; 328 pages (*out of print*)

No. 17 Directory of On-going Research in Cancer Epidemiology 1977
Edited by C.S. Muir and G. Wagner
1977; 599 pages (*out of print*)

No. 18 Environmental Carcinogens. Selected Methods of Analysis. Volume 1: Analysis of Volatile Nitrosamines in Food
Editor-in-Chief: H. Egan
1978; 212 pages (*out of print*)

Nó. 19 Environmental Aspects of N-Nitroso Compounds
Edited by E.A. Walker, M. Castegnaro, L. Griciute and R.E. Lyle
1978; 561 pages (*out of print*)

No. 20 Nasopharyngeal Carcinoma: Etiology and Control
Edited by G. de-Thé and Y. Ito
1978; 606 pages (*out of print*)

No. 21 Cancer Registration and its Techniques
Edited by R. MacLennan, C. Muir, R. Steinitz and A. Winkler
1978; 235 pages; £35.00

No. 22 Environmental Carcinogens. Selected Methods of Analysis. Volume 2: Methods for the Measurement of Vinyl Chloride in Poly(vinyl chloride), Air, Water and Foodstuffs
Editor-in-Chief: H. Egan
1978; 142 pages (*out of print*)

No. 23 Pathology of Tumours in Laboratory Animals. Volume II: Tumours of the Mouse
Editor-in-Chief: V.S. Turusov
1979; 669 pages (*out of print*)

Prices, valid for January 1990, are subject to change without notice

No. 24 **Oncogenesis and Herpesviruses III**
Edited by G. de-Thé, W. Henle and F. Rapp
1978; Part I: 580 pages, Part II: 512 pages (*out of print*)

No. 25 **Carcinogenic Risk. Strategies for Intervention**
Edited by W. Davis and C. Rosenfeld
1979; 280 pages (*out of print*)

No. 26 **Directory of On-going Research in Cancer Epidemiology 1978**
Edited by C.S. Muir and G. Wagner
1978; 550 pages (*out of print*)

No. 27 **Molecular and Cellular Aspects of Carcinogen Screening Tests**
Edited by R. Montesano, H. Bartsch and L. Tomatis
1980; 372 pages; £29.00

No. 28 **Directory of On-going Research in Cancer Epidemiology 1979**
Edited by C.S. Muir and G. Wagner
1979; 672 pages (*out of print*)

No. 29 **Environmental Carcinogens. Selected Methods of Analysis. Volume 3: Analysis of Polycyclic Aromatic Hydrocarbons in Environmental Samples**
Editor-in-Chief: H. Egan
1979; 240 pages (*out of print*)

No. 30 **Biological Effects of Mineral Fibres**
Editor-in-Chief: J.C. Wagner
1980; **Volume 1:** 494 pages; **Volume 2:** 513 pages; £65.00

No. 31 **N-Nitroso Compounds: Analysis, Formation and Occurrence**
Edited by E.A. Walker, L. Griciute, M. Castegnaro and M. Börzsönyi
1980; 835 pages (*out of print*)

No. 32 **Statistical Methods in Cancer Research. Volume 1. The Analysis of Case-control Studies**
By N.E. Breslow and N.E. Day
1980; 338 pages; £20.00

No. 33 **Handling Chemical Carcinogens in the Laboratory**
Edited by R. Montesano, *et al.*
1979; 32 pages (*out of print*)

No. 34 **Pathology of Tumours in Laboratory Animals. Volume III. Tumours of the Hamster**
Editor-in-Chief: V.S. Turusov
1982; 461 pages; £39.00

No. 35 **Directory of On-going Research in Cancer Epidemiology 1980**
Edited by C.S. Muir and G. Wagner
1980; 660 pages (*out of print*)

No. 36 **Cancer Mortality by Occupation and Social Class 1851-1971**
Edited by W.P.D. Logan
1982; 253 pages; £22.50

No. 37 **Laboratory Decontamination and Destruction of Aflatoxins B_1, B_2, G_1, G_2 in Laboratory Wastes**
Edited by M. Castegnaro, *et al.*
1980; 56 pages; £6.50

No. 38 **Directory of On-going Research in Cancer Epidemiology 1981**
Edited by C.S. Muir and G. Wagner
1981; 696 pages (*out of print*)

No. 39 **Host Factors in Human Carcinogenesis**
Edited by H. Bartsch and B. Armstrong
1982; 583 pages; £46.00

No. 40 **Environmental Carcinogens. Selected Methods of Analysis. Volume 4: Some Aromatic Amines and Azo Dyes in the General and Industrial Environment**
Edited by L. Fishbein, M. Castegnaro, I.K. O'Neill and H. Bartsch
1981; 347 pages; £29.00

No. 41 **N-Nitroso Compounds: Occurrence and Biological Effects**
Edited by H. Bartsch, I.K. O'Neill, M. Castegnaro and M. Okada
1982; 755 pages; £48.00

No. 42 **Cancer Incidence in Five Continents, Volume IV**
Edited by J. Waterhouse, C. Muir, K. Shanmugaratnam and J. Powell
1982; 811 pages (*out of print*)

No. 43 **Laboratory Decontamination and Destruction of Carcinogens in Laboratory Wastes: Some N-Nitrosamines**
Edited by M. Castegnaro, *et al.*
1982; 73 pages; £7.50

No. 44 **Environmental Carcinogens. Selected Methods of Analysis. Volume 5: Some Mycotoxins**
Edited by L. Stoloff, M. Castegnaro, P. Scott, I.K. O'Neill and H. Bartsch
1983; 455 pages; £29.00

No. 45 **Environmental Carcinogens. Selected Methods of Analysis. Volume 6: N-Nitroso Compounds**
Edited by R. Preussmann, I.K. O'Neill, G. Eisenbrand, B. Spiegelhalder and H. Bartsch
1983; 508 pages; £29.00

No. 46 **Directory of On-going Research in Cancer Epidemiology 1982**
Edited by C.S. Muir and G. Wagner
1982; 722 pages (*out of print*)

No. 47 **Cancer Incidence in Singapore 1968–1977**
Edited by K. Shanmugaratnam, H.P. Lee and N.E. Day
1983; 171 pages (*out of print*)

No. 48 **Cancer Incidence in the USSR (2nd Revised Edition)**
Edited by N.P. Napalkov, G.F. Tserkovny, V.M. Merabishvili, D.M. Parkin, M. Smans and C.S. Muir
1983; 75 pages; £12.00

No. 49 **Laboratory Decontamination and Destruction of Carcinogens in Laboratory Wastes: Some Polycyclic Aromatic Hydrocarbons**
Edited by M. Castegnaro, *et al.*
1983; 87 pages; £9.00

No. 50 **Directory of On-going Research in Cancer Epidemiology 1983**
Edited by C.S. Muir and G. Wagner
1983; 731 pages (*out of print*)

No. 51 **Modulators of Experimental Carcinogenesis**
Edited by V. Turusov and R. Montesano
1983; 307 pages; £22.50

No. 52 **Second Cancers in Relation to Radiation Treatment for Cervical Cancer: Results of a Cancer Registry Collaboration**
Edited by N.E. Day and J.C. Boice, Jr
1984; 207 pages; £20.00

No. 53 **Nickel in the Human Environment**
Editor-in-Chief: F.W. Sunderman, Jr
1984; 529 pages; £41.00

No. 54 **Laboratory Decontamination and Destruction of Carcinogens in Laboratory Wastes: Some Hydrazines**
Edited by M. Castegnaro, *et al.*
1983; 87 pages; £9.00

No. 55 **Laboratory Decontamination and Destruction of Carcinogens in Laboratory Wastes: Some N-Nitrosamines**
Edited by M. Castegnaro, *et al.*
1984; 66 pages; £7.50

No. 56 **Models, Mechanisms and Etiology of Tumour Promotion**
Edited by M. Börzsönyi, N.E. Day, K. Lapis and H. Yamasaki
1984; 532 pages; £42.00

No. 57 **N-Nitroso Compounds: Occurrence, Biological Effects and Relevance to Human Cancer**
Edited by I.K. O'Neill, R.C. von Borstel, C.T. Miller, J. Long and H. Bartsch
1984; 1013 pages; £80.00

No. 58 **Age-related Factors in Carcinogenesis**
Edited by A. Likhachev, V. Anisimov and R. Montesano
1985; 288 pages; £20.00

No. 59 **Monitoring Human Exposure to Carcinogenic and Mutagenic Agents**
Edited by A. Berlin, M. Draper, K. Hemminki and H. Vainio
1984; 457 pages; £27.50

No. 60 **Burkitt's Lymphoma: A Human Cancer Model**
Edited by G. Lenoir, G. O'Conor and C.L.M. Olweny
1985; 484 pages; £29.00

No. 61 **Laboratory Decontamination and Destruction of Carcinogens in Laboratory Wastes: Some Haloethers**
Edited by M. Castegnaro, *et al.*
1985; 55 pages; £7.50

No. 62 **Directory of On-going Research in Cancer Epidemiology 1984**
Edited by C.S. Muir and G. Wagner
1984; 717 pages (*out of print*)

No. 63 **Virus-associated Cancers in Africa**
Edited by A.O. Williams, G.T. O'Conor, G.B. de-Thé and C.A. Johnson
1984; 773 pages; £22.00

No. 64 **Laboratory Decontamination and Destruction of Carcinogens in Laboratory Wastes: Some Aromatic Amines and 4-Nitrobiphenyl**
Edited by M. Castegnaro, *et al.*
1985; 84 pages; £6.95

No. 65 **Interpretation of Negative Epidemiological Evidence for Carcinogenicity**
Edited by N.J. Wald and R. Doll
1985; 232 pages; £20.00

No. 66 **The Role of the Registry in Cancer Control**
Edited by D.M. Parkin, G. Wagner and C.S. Muir
1985; 152 pages; £10.00

No. 67 **Transformation Assay of Established Cell Lines: Mechanisms and Application**
Edited by T. Kakunaga and H. Yamasaki
1985; 225 pages; £20.00

No. 68 **Environmental Carcinogens. Selected Methods of Analysis. Volume 7. Some Volatile Halogenated Hydrocarbons**
Edited by L. Fishbein and I.K. O'Neill
1985; 479 pages; £42.00

No. 69 **Directory of On-going Research in Cancer Epidemiology 1985**
Edited by C.S. Muir and G. Wagner
1985; 745 pages; £22.00

No. 70 **The Role of Cyclic Nucleic Acid Adducts in Carcinogenesis and Mutagcnesis**
Edited by B. Singer and H. Bartsch
1986; 467 pages; £40.00

No. 71 **Environmental Carcinogens. Selected Methods of Analysis. Volume 8: Some Metals: As, Be, Cd, Cr, Ni, Pb, Se Zn**
Edited by I.K. O'Neill and, P. Schuller and L. Fishbein
1986; 485 pages; £42.00

No. 72 **Atlas of Cancer in Scotland, 1975–1980. Incidence and Epidemiological Perspective**
Edited by I. Kemp, P. Boyle, M. Smans and C.S. Muir
1985; 285 pages; £35.00

No. 73 **Laboratory Decontamination and Destruction of Carcinogens in Laboratory Wastes: Some Antineoplastic Agents**
Edited by M. Castegnaro, *et al.*
1985; 163 pages; £10.00

No. 74 **Tobacco: A Major International Health Hazard**
Edited by D. Zaridze and R. Peto
1986; 324 pages; £20.00

No. 75 **Cancer Occurrence in Developing Countries**
Edited by D.M. Parkin
1986; 339 pages; £20.00

No. 76 **Screening for Cancer of the Uterine Cervix**
Edited by M. Hakama, A.B. Miller and N.E. Day
1986; 315 pages; £25.00

No. 77 **Hexachlorobenzene: Proceedings of an International Symposium**
Edited by C.R. Morris and J.R.P. Cabral
1986; 668 pages; £50.00

No. 78 **Carcinogenicity of Alkylating Cytostatic Drugs**
Edited by D. Schmähl and J.M. Kaldor
1986; 337 pages; £25.00

No. 79 **Statistical Methods in Cancer Research. Volume III: The Design and Analsis of Long-term Animal Experiments**
Edited by J.J. Gart, D. Krewski, P.N. Lee, R.E. Tarone and J. Wahrendorf
1986; 213 pages; £20.00

No. 80 **Directory of On-going Research in Cancer Epidemiology 1986**
Edited by C.S. Muir and G. Wagner
1986; 805 pages; £22.00

No. 81 **Environmental Carcinogens: Methods of Analysis and Exposure Measurement. Volume 9: Passive Smoking**
Edited by I.K. O'Neill, K.D. Brunnemann, B. Dodet and D. Hoffmann
1987; 383 pages; £35.00

No. 82 **Statistical Methods in Cancer Research. Volume II: The Design and Analysis of Cohort Studies**
By N.E. Breslow and N.E. Day
1987; 404 pages; £30.00

No. 83 **Long-term and Short-term Assays for Carcinogens: A Critical Appraisal**
Edited by R. Montesano, H. Bartsch, H. Vainio, J. Wilbourn and H. Yamasaki
1986; 575 pages; £48.00

No. 84 **The Relevance of N-Nitroso Compounds to Human Cancer: Exposure and Mechanisms**
Edited by H. Bartsch, I.K. O'Neill and R. Schulte-Hermann
1987; 671 pages; £50.00

No. 85 **Environmental Carcinogens: Methods of Analysis and Exposure Measurement. Volume 10: Benzene and Alkylated Benzenes**
Edited by L. Fishbein and I.K. O'Neill
1988; 327 pages; £35.00

No. 86 **Directory of On-going Research in Cancer Epidemiology 1987**
Edited by D.M. Parkin and J. Wahrendorf
1987; 676 pages; £22.00

No. 87 **International Incidence of Childhood Cancer**
Edited by D.M. Parkin, C.A. Stiller, C.A. Bieber, G.J. Draper. B. Terracini and J.L. Young
1988; 401 pages; £35.00

No. 88 **Cancer Incidence in Five Continents Volume V**
Edited by C. Muir, J. Waterhouse, T. Mack, J. Powell and S. Whelan
1987; 1004 pages; £50.00

No. 89 **Method for Detecting DNA Damaging Agents in Humans: Applications in Cancer Epidemiology and Prevention**
Edited by H. Bartsch, K. Hemminki and I.K. O'Neill
1988; 518 pages; £45.00

No. 90 **Non-occupational Exposure to Mineral Fibres**
Edited by J. Bignon, J. Peto and R. Saracci
1989; 500 pages; £45.00

No. 91 **Trends in Cancer Incidence in Singapore 1968–1982**
Edited by H.P. Lee , N.E. Day and K. Shanmugaratnam
1988; 160 pages; £25.00

No. 92 **Cell Differentiation, Genes and Cancer**
Edited by T. Kakunaga, T. Sugimura, L. Tomatis and H. Yamasaki
1988; 204 pages; £25.00

No. 93 **Directory of On-going Research in Cancer Epidemiology 1988**
Edited by M. Coleman and J. Wahrendorf
1988; 662 pages (*out of print*)

No. 94 **Human Papillomavirus and Cervical Cancer**
Edited by N. Muñoz, F.X. Bosch and O.M.Jensen
1989; 154 pages; £19.00

No. 95 **Cancer Registration: Principles and Methods**
Edited by O.M. Jensen, D.M. Parkin, R. MacLennan, C.S. Muir and R. Skeet
Publ. due 1990; approx. 300 pages

No. 96 **Perinatal and Multigeneration Carcinogenesis**
Edited by N.P. Napalkov, J.M. Rice, L. Tomatis and H. Yamasaki
1989; 436 pages; £48.00

No. 97 **Occupational Exposure to Silica and Cancer Risk**
Edited by L. Simonato, A.C. Fletcher, R. Saracci and T. Thomas
1990; 124 pages; £19.00

No. 98 **Cancer Incidence in Jewish Migrants to Israel, 1961–1981**
Edited by R. Steinitz, D.M. Parkin, J.L. Young, C.A. Bieber and L. Katz
1989; 320 pages; £30.00

No. 99 **Pathology of Tumours in Laboratory Animals, Second Edition, Volume 1, Tumours of the Rat**
Edited by V.S. Turusov and U. Mohr
Publ. due 1990; 740 pages; £85.00

No. 100 **Cancer: Causes, Occurrence and Control**
Edited by L. Tomatis
1990; 352 pages; £24.00

No. 101 **Directory of On-going Research in Cancer Epidemiology 1989–90**
Edited by M. Coleman and J. Wahrendorf
1989; 818 pages; £36.00

No. 102 **Patterns of Cancer in Five Continents**
Edited by S.L. Whelan and D.M. Parkin
1990; 162 pages; £25.00

No. 103 **Evaluating Effectiveness of Primary Prevention of Cancer**
Edited by M. Hakama, V. Beral, J.W. Cullen and D.M. Parkin
Publ. due 1990; approx. 250 pages; £32.00

No. 104 **Complex Mixtures and Cancer Risk**
Edited by H. Vainio, M. Sorsa and A.J. McMichael
Publ. due 1990; 442 pages; £38.00

No. 105 **Relevance to Human Cancer of N-Nitroso Compounds, Tobacco Smoke and Mycotoxins**
Edited by I.K. O'Neill, J. Chen, S.H. Lu and H. Bartsch
Publ. due 1990; approx. 600 pages

IARC MONOGRAPHS ON THE EVALUATION OF CARCINOGENIC RISKS TO HUMANS

(Available from booksellers through the network of WHO Sales Agents*)

Volume 1 Some Inorganic Substances, Chlorinated Hydrocarbons, Aromatic Amines, N-nitroso Compounds, and Natural Products
1972; 184 pages (*out of print*)

Volume 2 Some Inorganic and Organometallic Compounds
1973; 181 pages (out of print)

Volume 3 Certain Polycyclic Aromatic Hydrocarbons and Heterocyclic Compounds
1973; 271 pages (*out of print*)

Volume 4 Some Aromatic Amines, Hydrazine and Related Substances, N-nitroso Compounds and Miscellaneous Alkylating Agents
1974; 286 pages;
Sw. fr. 18.-/US $14.40

Volume 5 Some Organochlorine Pesticides
1974; 241 pages (*out of print*)

Volume 6 Sex Hormones
1974; 243 pages (*out of print*)

Volume 7 Some Anti-Thyroid and Related Substances, Nitrofurans and Industrial Chemicals
1974; 326 pages (*out of print*)

Volume 8 Some Aromatic Azo Compounds
1975; 375 pages;
Sw. fr. 36.-/US $28.80

Volume 9 Some Aziridines, N-, S- and O-Mustards and Selenium
1975; 268 pages;
Sw.fr. 27.-/US $21.60

Volume 10 Some Naturally Occurring Substances
1976; 353 pages (*out of print*)

Volume 11 Cadmium, Nickel, Some Epoxides, Miscellaneous Industrial Chemicals and

General Considerations on Volatile Anaesthetics
1976; 306 pages (*out of print*)

Volume 12 Some Carbamates, Thiocarbamates and Carbazides
1976; 282 pages;
Sw fr. 34.-/US $27.20

Volume 13 Some Miscellaneous Pharmaceutical Substances
1977; 255 pages;
Sw. fr. 30.-/US$ 24.00

Volume 14 Asbestos
1977; 106 pages (*out of print*)

Volume 15 Some Fumigants, The Herbicides 2,4-D and 2,4,5-T, Chlorinated Dibenzodioxins and Miscellaneous Industrial Chemicals
1977; 354 pages;
Sw. fr. 50.-/US $40.00

Volume 16 Some Aromatic Amines and Related Nitro Compounds - Hair Dyes, Colouring Agents and Miscellaneous Industrial Chemicals
1978; 400 pages;
Sw. fr. 50.-/US $40.00

Volume 17 Some N-Nitroso Compounds
1987; 365 pages;
Sw. fr. 50.-/US $40.00

Volume 18 Polychlorinated Biphenyls and Polybrominated Biphenyls
1978; 140 pages;
Sw. fr. 20.-/US $16.00

Volume 19 Some Monomers, Plastics and Synthetic Elastomers, and Acrolein
1979; 513 pages;
Sw. fr. 60.-/US $48.00

Volume 20 Some Halogenated Hydrocarbons
1979; 609 pages (*out of print*)

Volume 21 Sex Hormones (II)
1979; 583 pages;
Sw. fr. 60.-/US $48.00

Volume 22 Some Non-Nutritive Sweetening Agents
1980; 208 pages;
Sw. fr. 25.-/US $20.00

Volume 23 Some Metals and Metallic Compounds
1980; 438 pages (*out of print*)

Volume 24 Some Pharmaceutical Drugs
1980; 337 pages;
Sw. fr. 40.-/US $32.00

Volume 25 Wood, Leather and Some Associated Industries
1981; 412 pages;
Sw. fr. 60-/US $48.00

Volume 26 Some Antineoplastic and Immunosuppressive Agents
1981; 411 pages;
Sw. fr. 62.-/US $49.60

Volume 27 Some Aromatic Amines, Anthraquinones and Nitroso Compounds, and Inorganic Fluorides Used in Drinking Water and Dental Preparations
1982; 341 pages;
Sw. fr. 40.-/US $32.00

Volume 28 The Rubber Industry
1982; 486 pages;
Sw. fr. 70.-/US $56.00

Volume 29 Some Industrial Chemicals and Dyestuffs
1982; 416 pages;
Sw. fr. 60.-/US $48.00

Volume 30 **Miscellaneous Pesticides**
1983; 424 pages;
Sw. fr. 60.-/US $48.00

Volume 31 **Some Food Additives, Feed Additives and Naturally Occurring Substances**
1983; 314 pages;
Sw. fr. 60-/US $48.00

Volume 32 **Polynuclear Aromatic Compounds, Part 1: Chemical, Environmental and Experimental Data**
1984; 477 pages;
Sw. fr. 60.-/US $48.00

Volume 33 **Polynuclear Aromatic Compounds, Part 2: Carbon Blacks, Mineral Oils and Some Nitroarenes**
1984; 245 pages;
Sw. fr. 50.-/US $40.00

Volume 34 **Polynuclear Aromatic Compounds, Part 3: Industrial Exposures in Aluminium Production, Coal Gasification, Coke Production, and Iron and Steel Founding**
1984; 219 pages;
Sw. fr. 48.-/US $38.40

Volume 35 **Polynuclear Aromatic Compounds: Part 4: Bitumens, Coal-Tars and Derived Products, Shale-Oils and Soots**
1985; 271 pages;
Sw. fr. 70.-/US $56.00

Volume 37 **Tobacco Habits Other than Smoking: Betel-Quid and Areca-Nut Chewing; and some Related Nitrosamines**
1985; 291 pages;
Sw. fr. 70.-/US $56.00

Volume 38 **Tobacco Smoking**
1986; 421 pages;
Sw. fr. 75.-/US $60.00

Volume 39 **Some Chemicals Used in Plastics and Elastomers**
1986; 403 pages;
Sw. fr. 60.-/US $48.00

Volume 40 **Some Naturally Occurring and Synthetic Food Components, Furocoumarins and Ultraviolet Radiation**
1986; 444 pages;
Sw. fr. 65.-/US $52.00

Volume 41 **Some Halogenated Hydrocarbons and Pesticide Exposures**
1986; 434 pages;
Sw. fr. 65.-/US $52.00

Volume 42 **Silica and Some Silicates**
1987; 289 pages;
Sw. fr. 65.-/US $52.00

Volume 43 **Man-Made Mineral Fibres and Radon**
1988; 300 pages;
Sw. fr. 65.-/US $52.00

Volume 44 **Alcohol Drinking**
1988; 416 pages;
Sw. fr. 65.-/US $52.00

Volume 45 **Occupational Exposures in Petroleum Refining; Crude Oil and Major Petroleum Fuels**
1989; 322 pages;
Sw. fr. 65.-/US $52.00

Volume 46 **Diesel and Gasoline Engine Exhausts and Some Nitroarenes**
1989; 458 pages;
Sw. fr. 65.-/US $52.00

Volume 47 **Some Organic Solvents, Resin Monomers and Related Compounds, Pigments and Occupational Exposures in Paint Manufacture and Painting**
1990; 536 pages;
Sw. fr. 85.-/US $68.00

Volume 48 **Some Flame Retardants and Textile Chemicals, and Exposures in the Textile Manufacturing Industry**
1990; 345 pages;
Sw. fr. 65.-/US $52.00

Supplement No. 1
Chemicals and Industrial Processes Associated with Cancer in Humans (IARC Monographs, Volumes 1 to 20)
1979; 71 pages; (*out of print*)

Supplement No. 2
Long-Term and Short-Term Screening Assays for Carcinogens: A Critical Appraisal
1980; 426 pages;
Sw. fr. 40.-/US $32.00

Supplement No. 3
Cross Index of Synonyms and Trade Names in Volumes 1 to 26
1982; 199 pages (*out of print*)

Supplement No. 4
Chemicals, Industrial Processes and Industries Associated with Cancer in Humans (IARC Monographs, Volumes 1 to 29)
1982; 292 pages (*out of print*)

Supplement No. 5
Cross Index of Synonyms and Trade Names in Volumes 1 to 36
1985; 259 pages;
Sw. fr. 46.-/US $36.80

Supplement No. 6
Genetic and Related Effects: An Updating of Selected IARC Monographs from Volumes 1 to 42
1987; 729 pages;
Sw. fr. 80.-/US $64.00

Supplement No. 7
Overall Evaluations of Carcinogenicity: An Updating of IARC Monographs Volumes 1-42
1987; 434 pages;
Sw. fr. 65.-/US $52.00

Supplement No. 8
Cross Index of Synonyms and Trade Names in Volumes 1 to 46 of the IARC Monographs
Publ. 1990; 260 pages;
Sw. fr. 60.-/US $48.00

IARC TECHNICAL REPORTS*

No. 1 **Cancer in Costa Rica**
Edited by R. Sierra,
R. Barrantes, G. Muñoz Leiva,
D.M. Parkin, C.A. Bieber and
N. Muñoz Calero
1988; 124 pages;
Sw. fr. 30.-/US $24.00

No. 2 **SEARCH: A Computer Package to Assist the Statistical Analysis of Case-Control Studies**
Edited by G.J. Macfarlane,
P. Boyle and P. Maisonneuve (in press)

No. 3 **Cancer Registration in the European Economic Community**
Edited by M.P. Coleman and
E. Démaret
1988; 188 pages;
Sw. fr. 30.-/US $24.00

No. 4 **Diet, Hormones and Cancer: Methodological Issues for Prospective Studies**
Edited by E. Riboli and
R. Saracci
1988; 156 pages;
Sw. fr. 30.-/US $24.00

No. 5 **Cancer in the Philippines**
Edited by A.V. Laudico,
D. Esteban and D.M. Parkin
1989; 186 pages;
Sw. fr. 30.-/US $24.00

No. 6 **La genèse du Centre International de Recherche sur le Cancer**
Par R. Sohier et A.G.B. Sutherland
1990; 104 pages
Sw. fr. 30.-/US $24.00

No. 7 **Epidémiologie du cancer dans les pays de langue latine**
1990; 310 pages
Sw. fr. 30.-/US $24.00

No. 8 **Comparative Study of Anti-Smoking Legislation in Countries of the European Economic Community**
Edited by A. Sasco
1990; c. 80 pages
Sw. fr. 30.-/US $24.00
(English and French editions available)

DIRECTORY OF CHEMICALS BEING TESTED FOR CARCINOGENICITY
(Until Vol. 13 Information Bulletin on the Survey of Chemicals Being Tested for Carcinogenicity)*

No. 8 **Edited by M.-J. Ghess, H. Bartsch and L. Tomatis**
1979; 604 pages; Sw. fr. 40.-

No. 9 **Edited by M.-J. Ghess, J.D. Wilbourn, H. Bartsch and L. Tomatis**
1981; 294 pages; Sw. fr. 41.-

No. 10 **Edited by M.-J. Ghess, J.D. Wilbourn and H. Bartsch**
1982; 362 pages; Sw. fr. 42.-

No. 11 **Edited by M.-J. Ghess, J.D. Wilbourn, H. Vainio and H. Bartsch**
1984; 362 pages; Sw. fr. 50.-

No. 12 **Edited by M.-J. Ghess, J.D. Wilbourn, A. Tossavainen and H. Vainio**
1986; 385 pages; Sw. fr. 50.-

No. 13 **Edited by M.-J. Ghess, J.D. Wilbourn and A. Aitio**
1988; 404 pages; Sw. fr. 43.-

No. 14 **Edited by M.-J. Ghess, J.D. Wilbourn and H. Vainio**
1990; c. 400 pages;
Sw. fr. 45.-

NON-SERIAL PUBLICATIONS †

Alcool et Cancer
By A. Tuyns (in French only)
1978; 42 pages; Fr. fr. 35.-

Cancer Morbidity and Causes of Death Among Danish Brewery Workers
By O.M. Jensen 1980;
143 pages; Fr. fr. 75.-

Directory of Computer Systems Used in Cancer Registries
By H.R. Menck and D.M. Parkin 1986; 236 pages;
Fr. fr. 50.-

* Available from booksellers through the network of WHO sales agents.

†Available directly from IARC